Loo Rolls to Lycra

Loo Rolls to Lycra

The Ironman Dreams of an IBD Sufferer

Caroline Bramwell

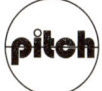

First published by Pitch Publishing, 2018

Pitch Publishing
A2 Yeoman Gate
Yeoman Way
Worthing
Sussex
BN13 3QZ
www.pitchpublishing.co.uk
info@pitchpublishing.co.uk

© 2018, Caroline Bramwell

Every effort has been made to trace the copyright.
Any oversight will be rectified in future editions at the
earliest opportunity by the publisher.

All rights reserved. No part of this book may be reproduced,
sold or utilised in any form or transmitted in any form or by
any means, electronic or mechanical, including photocopying,
recording or by any information storage and retrieval system,
without prior permission in writing from the Publisher.

A CIP catalogue record is available for this book
from the British Library.

ISBN 978-1-78531-350-9

Typesetting and origination by Pitch Publishing
Printed in the UK by TJ International, Cornwall

Contents

Chapter One 9

Chapter Two 28

Chapter Three 40

Chapter Four 50

Chapter Five 66

Chapter Six 73

Chapter Seven 88

Chapter Eight 104

Chapter Nine 117

Chapter Ten 129

Chapter Eleven 145

Chapter Twelve 157

Chapter Thirteen 174

Chapter Fourteen 193

Chapter Fifteen 208

Dedication

To Craig for being there through the tough times that my medicated brain cannot remember

To Robert and Natasha for being my inspiration to get fit and become a triathlete

To my mum and sisters for always encouraging me

To Dad – always love you, always miss you

Chapter One

'HOW MUCH longer are you going to be? Someone's going to spot us!'

As my husband acted as lookout on the roadside, trying to be as inconspicuous as possible, I was crouched as low as I could behind the decorative flower bed on one of the busiest main roads in Barnstaple at prime time on a Saturday evening. There wasn't anything I could do; this, for me, was a normal occurrence. As I squatted uncomfortably amongst the bushes with my back up against a small, cold brick wall, I was in so much pain and my body was turning itself inside out. Thankfully the darkness helped to obscure the sight of me hunkering down like a common tramp in the undergrowth. This flower bed had been the nearest location that I could find to dive into when my ulcerative colitis attack came on; next to the pay meter of a car park, I was hoping against all odds that, at 11pm, no one was going to be needing a car park ticket!

When my husband, Craig, had called out those words in hushed tones – 'How much longer are you going to be?' – I'd had to bite my tongue. 'I didn't exactly think about timing myself,' was the retort in my head. From the aching in my legs I knew I'd been here a long time – maybe up to 30 minutes? Or maybe it had been longer? I can imagine for him, loitering on the roadside, he'd probably looked a bit suspect as well as being bored out of his mind. Who would want to stand on the street as a lookout after a night out?

I was in a whole different world of pain, one that I'd come to live with over the last five years. I would much rather be the embarrassed lookout, trying to distract the passers-by with a cheery 'Good evening', than being the anxious and distraught person that I now was, hiding in the bushes.

The evening had started out so well. It was a rare thing to get an evening out together, partly due to my illness and partly because we didn't often manage to get a babysitter. So we'd planned to go to the cinema. Nothing strenuous – just a lovely 'grown-ups' evening to see the latest blockbuster. I'd planned my day carefully so that I hadn't eaten anything that might upset my stomach; I'd kept the day as stress-free as possible and it was all paying off. I'd managed a whole evening without incident – watching the whole film without having to dash off at regular intervals to the toilet. For once, I'd been feeling like a normal human being again as we watched the final film credits roll. The biggest incident of the evening was me kicking over a huge carton of sticky sweet popcorn that even the cinema attendant came and swept up with a huff.

As we left the cinema for the short walk to the car park, my stomach started to cramp up. 'Oh no, not now!' I thought; I turned to Craig, who could see by the worried look on my face that I was having a problem. I had to

ONE

find somewhere to go, right this second! These attacks are instant, and I mean *really* instant! We had already walked past the only pub near the car park, and I'd never make it back there in time anyway. Approaching the car park, my only option was the bushes. They weren't exactly big bushes to hide behind, but it was that or nothing!

So, how does a grown woman in her early 40s stoop so low as to be crouching in the bushes?

The last four years have been a living hell ... to be honest, it really all started when I was pregnant with my daughter, Natasha.

* * * * *

It's October 2004 and I am three months pregnant with my second child; I'm a nervous mum-to-be. Since my son, Robert, was born just over a year ago, I've sadly had two miscarriages, so this time I've been extremely cautious and tried to make sure my life has been calm and stress-free. In the bathroom for the usual 'morning ablutions', I am therefore immediately panicked at the sight of blood in the toilet bowl. 'Please, no, not again.'

A mother's instinct kicks in and I immediately get myself an appointment with my GP. However, it's not right – it's not like before. The bleeding isn't coming from the pregnancy. That's a relief, but it leaves some unanswered questions about what this really is. The doctor wants to monitor things – if she's got any ideas, she's definitely not prepared to share them with me at the moment.

As the weeks pass and the baby inside me continues to grow, the bleeding and upset stomach doesn't let up. Clearly there is something else going on, as I am spending longer in the toilet. At first it's suggested that it could be irritable bowel syndrome (IBS), but from the way in which I explain to her that I get a slight urgency for going to the toilet, the doctor suspects that it could be ulcerative colitis. I've never heard of ulcerative colitis, and I've no idea what causes it or how it's cured. Until we know for sure, the doctor cannot make a confirmed diagnosis. The only way we are going to know for sure is with an internal inspection – a colonoscopy – but this could put the baby at risk of miscarriage, so we have to leave it until all risk to the baby has passed.

At seven months pregnant, the decision is made to carry out the internal investigation. At the hospital, I am asked to drink a glutinous concoction that both looks and tastes like thick, gritty mud. It smells disgusting, and in order to swallow it, I have to hold my nose. This is so gross. This foul-smelling swamp sludge is supposedly going to 'clear me out'. I'm left in a small private room with an en-suite toilet, and I sit and wait. It doesn't take long to work. Oh my word, I dash to the toilet and my body drains itself at full pelt! After two further dashes to the toilet, my body feels racked and empty.

Nervously, dressed in an unglamorous blue hospital gown, loosely tied down the back to provide some modesty, I feel very exposed both physically and mentally. A gently spoken nurse comes in to see if I'm OK and tells me it's time to go through to the next room, where the consultant will carry out the procedure. I lie down on the table and the consultant explains to me what is going to happen. The camera is going to be passed up my back passage and around the bend that is the sigmoid. He's going to be looking for signs of inflammation, which, if I want, I can see on the television screen beside the table.

I roll over with my bum exposed, counterbalanced by my baby bump, which is nestled in the drapes of the

ONE

blue gown. With three people in the room, this feels like a performance in embarrassment. But it's got to be done. As the consultant talks to me throughout, the procedure isn't too bad until it meets the sigmoid. As this point, the camera has to go around a bend, which becomes exceedingly uncomfortable. I wince at the sudden pain and discomfort, and I'm asked to move my body a little to ease it going through. It's as far as it's going to need to go, and on the end of the instrument is a small 'grabber' that takes a biopsy. We can all see on the screen that the lining of my bowel is red and inflamed. It's confirmed that I have ulcerative colitis (UC).

Ulcerative colitis is an autoimmune disorder, sometimes thought to be hereditary, but that's not always the case. It's definitely not something that runs in my family. In essence, your body's natural defence mechanism will fight off viruses, but with Crohn's disease or colitis the body's defence system thinks you are the virus, so it attacks your intestine. By attacking the lining of the intestine, this becomes ulcerated and bleeds, which was the first indicator for me. But it's not just that the intestine is ulcerated – simply eating can keep it aggravated. It was explained to me that it's like having an open wound on your skin and constantly rubbing food and dirt over it; it's not likely to heal when it's constantly being rubbed.

* * * * *

Natasha is born by caesarean, as she ended up refusing to turn around, so her head was high and her feet were pushing downwards. If it wasn't bad enough having to need the loo with my UC, I've also had her kicking my bladder, making me need to pee all the time as well through the later stages of pregnancy. The hospital did try turning her with acupuncture, but she was stubborn and wouldn't shift.

As Craig watches on, the nurse lifts our beautiful baby girl up for me to see and I hold her close. I may have had to put up with tummy upsets whilst pregnant, but this little bundle is so worth all the aggravation.

Discharged within the week, I'm home with Craig and my toddler, Robert, and now we have our final member of the family all tucked up with us. Recovering from the caesarean will take a few weeks, but it feels great to be home in my own bed with Natasha in the crib beside it. I've been breastfeeding her from the moment she was born, but as we move into the second week at home she is in need of more bottle feeding. I expect to be losing some of the weight that I've carried whilst I was pregnant, but after the initial drop it continues to fall. Whilst I feel like I am getting back into shape, this is just far too rapid.

As I get thinner by the day, I am struggling to produce enough milk to feed Natasha; my body is failing me as a mother. This disease is now starting to take over my body. Whilst I was carrying the baby, I felt like I was battling to protect her – but, since she was safely delivered, this disease has had free rein to really have an impact on me. The ulceration in my colon is making blood loss a regular occurrence, and with this comes fatigue.

When the lining of the intestine is so inflamed and bleeding, the knock-on effect is twofold. There is the effect of fatigue simply due to the amount of blood loss, but also the body is unable to absorb enough nutrients from the food I'm eating, because this is absorbed through the lining of the intestine. So it's a double whammy of a downward spiral. Within two weeks of giving birth to Natasha, I have lost two stone in weight; and with the

ONE

exhaustion of the disease, I need to rest more and more. With Robert not yet two years old and now with baby Natasha, Craig takes charge of doing all the night feeds for Natasha with the bottles I've prepared.

My doctor refers me to a specialist consultant at North Devon District Hospital – the same man who carried out the sigmoidoscopy on me just a few short months ago. His very matter-of-fact approach is harsh, but I guess he's being a realist. This is a disease, not just a condition that can be cured with a course of tablets. The only way to stop my body from attacking itself is to suppress the autoimmune system: to turn off that defence mechanism that has gone awry and normally protects our bodies. This entails some lengthy discussions about steroids.

'Steroids? Aren't they bad for you? Don't they have side effects?'

'Yes, there are side effects,' the consultant admits, 'but we will give you some tablets to counteract those.'

To begin with, he prescribes for me some prednisolone, a topical steroid foam. The plan is to use this on a regular basis at the point of the problem, to try to calm down the inflammation. I am to try it for a few weeks and see how it improves things. I pick up the bulky plain paper bag from the dispensary in the hospital, now feeling armed with my own defence mechanism against this disease. To say that using this for the first time was a unique experience is an understatement. The bag contained a canister of foam and a large quantity of plastic straws. It doesn't take much imagination to realise how this is going to get to the point of delivery! I've squatted over a few unpleasant toilets on foreign holidays in my time, but trying to 'squat and squirt' would put the skills of a contortionist to the test.

After a few weeks, the foam isn't having much effect, except perhaps I'm walking slightly differently! So it's a repeat visit to the consultant for an update. Clearly this disease has got a better grip on my gut than I have, so we have to look at upping the steroids in my body to battle this. We need to find a balance between keeping the disease under control and not overloading my body with unnecessary steroids, as there is only a certain limit we can go to based on my weight. So the decision is made to give me a relatively low level of steroids in tablet form, as well as the foam, for the time being. The steroids, however, can cause osteoarthritis and have other nasty effects on your internal organs, so I am prescribed a concoction of medication for each to treat the effects of the other. This includes taking ferrous sulphate (iron tablets) and calcium tablets.

As things start to settle down, with less and less bleeding, I'm at last starting to feel normal again and feel like we've got this under control. After all, when you're ill with anything, it takes time to recover and start getting back to your old self. I am, however, a little concerned at having to be on the steroids, and I know the idea is to get things under control now, then wean down the steroids so my body can cope on its own again.

* * * * *

It's taken me several months to feel like I'm at the point of reducing the steroid dosage, and I'll admit I'm a little bit nervous – and excited at the same time – to be dropping this. There's a bit of me that wants to get rid of the steroids altogether, but I know that's not going to be possible at the moment. By going 'cold turkey', my body, which has become dependent on the tablets to keep my immune

ONE

system suppressed, won't be able to cope so suddenly, and I know the flare-up from the ulcerative colitis will be so much worse. So this is a gentle reduction of steroids, giving my body time to 'rebalance' itself.

With the flare-ups more manageable, being a mum again is a wonderful feeling, and I plan a trip into Barnstaple for some clothes shopping with Natasha. She's not yet a year old, so having her baby buggy makes it so much easier for me to carry more purchases, and means I don't have to carry her. Ulcerative colitis is a very unpredictable disease. Whilst the condition eats away at your insides, as it progresses it is causing me to have some 'urgent' toilet visits. I don't mean like someone who just feels that they really desperately need the toilet; most people can hang on until they find a loo. But with ulcerative colitis you lose even that control. The only way to describe it is like having food poisoning but without the sickness.

Browsing amongst the rails of gorgeous baby clothes in Mothercare, my stomach suddenly starts to cramp up. Panic-stricken, I look around to see if they've got any customer toilets in the store. Unfortunately, not being a large store, they don't! Terrified of what is about to happen right here in the middle of the store, I ask the girl on the checkout if they have a toilet I could use urgently.

'I'm very sorry, we don't have customer toilets. The nearest public toilets are down the other end of the shopping centre,' she says, pointing out of the store.

'I won't make it that far!' I cry. 'I've got a medical condition called ulcerative colitis, which means when I need to go, I need to go immediately. If I don't get to a toilet straight away, I'm going to be in an awful mess. It's pretty much uncontrollable.'

Seeing my distress, the manager standing beside the young sales assistant spots that there's a problem and immediately steps in to help.

'We do have our staff toilet out the back, which you can use. However, you won't be able to get the buggy in there with you, it's just a tiny toilet. But don't worry, we will look after your daughter here behind the counter while you use the toilet.'

I cannot thank her enough, although the thought of leaving my baby daughter behind the counter in the shop, whilst I am out the back, terrifies me. I'm led to the back of the shop and out through their warehouse to a tiny toilet cubicle – really it's just the size of a cupboard. I dash in, lock the door and burst into floods of tears. 'I hate this disease – why me?' I sob.

After about 20 minutes of pain and suffering, I make my way back to the shop floor. Natasha is happily dozing in her buggy, oblivious to the disappearance of her distraught mother. The manager and shop assistant are wonderfully kind and ask if I'm OK. Now that the urgency has passed, I am able to explain to them more about the disease and the impact it has on my body. I cannot say thank you enough to them for their consideration and help. Their understanding means a great deal to me. I count myself lucky that I was in Mothercare when this attack happened; if I'd been in a hardware store or a large supermarket, would they have been so considerate to a mum in distress? Would they have done the same thing? I'd like to think so.

After this terrible episode, I vow never to go shopping with my children alone; Craig is going to have to come with me in case it happens again. And happen again, it does! In fact, it increasingly becomes a problem. For

ONE

months, the urgent attacks come on. At first they are just intermittent and it's difficult to pinpoint what causes them. Often it's just picking something up and putting a strain on my stomach, or it could be having a stressful day. Irritable bowel syndrome is brought on by anxiety and lifestyle stresses, but this inflammatory bowel disease (IBD) is different.

Sadly, people do get the two conditions confused. So often it is thought by friends and family that IBD is the same as IBS and that I should just 'take it a bit easy'. I can't take life easy with an 18-month-old and a 3-year-old. When the children are crawling around on the floor in the lounge, I get down to join in, but simply the movement of rolling around on the floor causes the cramping pain, which signals having to make an emergency dash to the toilet. As I come to identify what might trigger an attack, the more I hold back. I can no longer get down on the floor and play with the children, I can no longer pick them up and swing them around, I can no longer take them to the park to play, where there are no toilets nearby. This horrible disease is stopping me from doing all the things a mum and dad do with their kids in these early formative years. It becomes heartbreaking to watch Craig play with Robert and Natasha in a way that I want to, to throw myself into being an active, fun-loving mum, as I was when Robert was born.

Shopping trips into town become a regular family event now, and with the increasing number of attacks I am getting, my steroid dosage is having to be increased just to keep the condition under control. This doesn't mean it stops the bouts of urgency – it just tries to limit them. My life is now being controlled by toilets. I can't go anywhere where there isn't a toilet, and I even consider applying for a Blue Badge. This would entitle me to park up on double yellow lines, or in disabled car-parking bays, which would be close to a loo in case of emergency. But I don't consider myself to be 'disabled' in the way anyone would traditionally consider 'disabled' to mean. So I choose not to apply for the Badge. I do, however, become a member of Crohn's & Colitis UK, who, with their welcome pack, send me a Radar key and a 'Can't Wait Card', which I can show someone if I am in a mad rush for the toilet, without having to explain it all. The Radar key looks like a giant key to some magical Pandora's box – maybe, in a way, it is. It will allow me access to disabled toilets.

However, having such a 'magical' key that gives me access to the inner sanctum of a large disabled toilet facility, especially when I have two small children in tow, brought its own issues. You see, when someone sees me coming out of the disabled toilet with two small children, I'll get stared at and even have remarks made to me along the lines of, 'This is for disabled people, it's not for families.' Whilst I want to snap back at the individual, I have to take a deep breath and explain calmly that I have a medical condition. Of course, being a condition about bowels and pooing, most people feel very uncomfortable and embarrassed at having asked. Maybe next time they won't be so quick to judge.

So, on trips to the big shopping centre in town, to save myself the embarrassment of people questioning my right to use the disabled toilets, and holding up others, I generally endeavour to use the regular ladies' toilets. I might be in there for ages. The urgency comes on so fast, and my body starts to empty so fast, just like when I took that swamp sludge for the sigmoidoscopy. But this time, it won't stop. My body cramps up, trying to excrete everything it

ONE

contains and more; it's an involuntary spasming that leaves my stomach aching, as though a tight band has been put around my body and tightened and tightened until I hurt. Poor Craig and the children are left outside waiting for half an hour or more for me to reappear – a washed-out, frail version of the me that went in.

On one occasion, I take Natasha into the ladies' toilets to change her nappy. Laid out on the fold-down changing board, with the little straps that hold the wriggly little person in one place, I've just taken off her nappy when the cramping starts. Now I've got a big dilemma: Natasha's halfway through a nappy change in the middle of the toilets and I'm about to poo myself! I ask one of the ladies queuing for the toilets to quickly go and call my husband, who is waiting outside. Startled, she does as I ask, and Craig, with Robert in tow, has to come through into the ladies' toilets to pick up where I am about to have to leave off. Apologising profusely to the women queuing for the toilets, Craig takes over the nappy change, whilst I dash for the first available cubicle, queue-jumping in the process whilst Craig explains what the problem is.

From that point on, Craig becomes the nappy-changer on every outing. His role becomes that of mum and dad rolled into one. Neither of us can trust my body to behave in any situation, so, rather than having the same problem happening again, it seems simpler for Craig to deal with Natasha, as more often than not I'll need the toilet and be gone for quite some time.

* * * * *

As I'm on increasingly higher dosages of steroids, the doctor and hospital consultant are having to monitor how my body is coping with all these drugs. The steroids have a bad effect on my internal organs, so I have to take extra drugs to counteract that effect. Plus I have to be careful in the sun, as the steroids thin the skin. But in order to know how much of each drug I should have so that it isn't having a detrimental effect on my internal organs, I have to get blood samples taken every two weeks. Each visit, I have to switch from my left arm to my right to preserve the integrity of my veins, and if the needle doesn't go in easily, I end up with terrible bruising in my arm, making me look like some kind of drug addict.

Taking my bloods is routine for me, and as Natasha and Robert are growing up and come with me to my doctor appointments, they are fascinated by the whole process. I don't want my children to grow up worrying about needles, so they get 'hands on' and get to hold the phial after it's been filled, amazed at how it feels warm in their little hands.

Living with a disease like this, your whole life revolves around medication, blood tests, toilets and hospital appointments. My stomach becomes bloated quite frequently, and I find that this can make my urgent dash to the toilet more volatile. Looking online for information, I can only find forums full of other people who have the condition and it's all 'woe is me'. The stories of their illness and how bad they feel, and how they cannot do anything, are really depressing, and the thought that this is how life is going to be for me is a bleak prospect.

Thinking that there must be some natural remedies for this condition, I've read up that wheat and dairy can aggravate the gut, so cutting these out could help. I've also come across Aloe Vera, which you can take in a drink form. It tastes pretty foul to me, but as aloe is a natural healer, the concept is that this lines the inside of your

ONE

intestine. I'm not sure exactly how effective this can be, and as my condition worsens it is definitely not having any effect. I think my system is beyond the point of being gently healed by a plant drink.

Changing my diet, however, does seem to have a calming effect on my system. By cutting out bread, I'm getting less bloating. The bloating has become an increasingly big part of this condition. It's been terribly depressing seeing myself ballooning up, not just from my gut feeling swollen and uncomfortable, but also with the side effects of the increasing dosage of steroids. Over time I have begun to look like I've been pumped up like a helium balloon; I've now got what is called 'moon face' – my face has puffed up and it's no longer me looking back from the mirror in the morning. My clothes no longer fit me, and I am having to wear my dark, loose pregnancy outfits again. To be honest, I actually look pregnant again. I avoid looking in a mirror as much as possible now, as it just makes me cry to see myself looking so huge. My eyes look like slits in my big, inflated face. This is the drugs taking full impact on my body. I have no choice but to take the tablets, hence my desperate endeavours to find natural remedies to help manage this condition so I can come off the medication.

Cutting out bread is easy – just stop eating sandwiches – but it's actually going gluten-free that seems to calm my system the most. So this means finding alternatives to eat. I've bought myself a bread maker and spelt flour, and I've started to make my own spelt bread. Being an ancient form of wheat, I have found it doesn't create the gluten issues of more common wheat. I've also found a little local bakery that makes fresh rye bread, which has also been a great alternative to the bread I used to eat, as this hasn't caused me any bloating. But going gluten-free isn't just about bread: I have to cut out all forms of gluten, and I've now become obsessed with checking the details on the packets of everything we buy. No pastry, no gravy … it's shocking how much of our everyday food contains gluten. Endeavouring to go gluten-free and dairy-free at the same time is doubly tough, and my choice of foods is dwindling to a very slim range. I'm sure I'm not getting the best nutrient intake.

Craig has pretty much taken over the running of the house and kids, including cooking dinners every evening. However, he's having to create different meals for me every night, and it's just more for him to have to cope with.

I've taken to juicing wheatgrass. I've bought a juicer, which you clamp on to the side of your kitchen unit and then grind the grass through it to get the juice. It's a laborious task for such a small amount of juice from all the effort. The house is now also looking like a garden centre, as I've taken to ordering trays of growing wheatgrass on a regular basis. The only place where I can keep it is in the conservatory which adjoins our kitchen. I can easily access it for my juicing. Craig thinks it's all getting a little extreme, but I'm trying everything.

Talking to my consultant at the hospital, I explain to him what I'm doing with my diet. He tells me that food has nothing to do with it. But I know my own body, and I know that with cutting out the gluten, in particular, I'm feeling less bloated and uncomfortable and therefore not dashing to the toilet quite so much.

Craig's being mum and dad these days, because I'm simply unable to cope. The steroids are really messing with my head; it's like there's loads of 'noise' going on all

ONE

the time inside my head and I cannot think straight. Craig and I run our own PR, marketing and graphic design business, which I'm the 'front man' for; if I don't go out and look for new work, then there's nothing new coming in to keep us busy or pay the wages. But I'm struggling at the office with fatigue and what I call my 'noisy head'. Up until now we have employed two staff – one is an account executive and the other is my office manager, who looks after the accounts too – but it's worrying that I cannot bring in new work and I am increasingly having to have a quiet time to take a power nap in the afternoon in the office, whilst the others 'man the fort'.

Craig and I decide that I should just focus on the business and not worry about the house and kids, after an incident at Tesco one Saturday morning. I take Robert and Natasha with me for our regular weekly shop at the supermarket. Parked up in the 'mother and toddler' bay, I load the two of them into the double seats in the front of the shopping trolley and head into the store, armed with my long list of groceries and household stuff. The store is busy; I've picked a bad time to come – mid-morning on a Saturday. I head up and down the first two aisles of fruit and vegetables, looking at my list to make sure I haven't forgotten anything. Trying to get around the top of the aisle into the next one, there's always a bottleneck of trollies and people. Why do people find it necessary to leave their trolley unattended in places where people are coming round, whilst they wander off to pick an item off the opposite aisle? This really irritates me. The next aisle is equally busy with families; feeling my frustration starting to bubble up, my head is starting to spin and I cannot seem to concentrate. Now there are two men chatting in the middle of the aisle, totally oblivious to the fact that their trollies have completely blocked the aisle and no one can get through.

With a sharp 'Excuse me', I glare at the men as I barge my way through them, bumping one of the trollies out of the way as I go. I'm not someone who would ever get angry at something so minor, but I am absolutely seething. Inside my head I am screaming; my children keep grabbing items from the trolley behind them, thinking it's a great game, but I cannot think; my heart's racing; I've got to get out of here!

Pushing the trolley to the front of the store to where I see a shop assistant, I grab both the children out of their seats and sob to the lady, 'I can't do this, it's just too much. I'll have to come back when it's not busy.' Leaving this startled young lady with a half-loaded trolley, I dash out to the car, strap the children into their car seats and ring home, crying my eyes out. I cannot even cope with going food shopping now, and all this upset has set my stomach off into cramping again. Thankfully I don't live far away, and Craig comes out to help me bring the children in whilst I dash to the toilet. Another disastrous attempt to be a normal mum has ended with me back in the toilet again.

So now, I don't take the children out into town on my own, I cannot play with them on the floor and I cannot even go supermarket shopping. Hence the decision that Craig should take control of all this for me, so I can at least attempt to focus on work.

Craig, however, is having to contend with another side effect of my steroids. Usually a placid, friendly person, I have always been prone to sleepwalking. But now even this has been pushed to extremes with this harsh medication. In the middle of the night, without warning,

ONE

I am sitting up in bed, and punching Craig in the head and swearing. Who is this monster? I only find out the following morning, when I see Craig has a yellow eye from where I've punched him in the face. I have absolutely no recollection whatsoever of doing this, and that's upsetting. If I could do this to my husband, what else might I do in my sleep?

It isn't too long before we find out. Late one evening whilst Craig is up watching a movie, he hears me coming down the stairs. He calls out, and I clearly don't respond, so he's a little concerned. Following me into the back office, he rapidly snatches the telephone out of my hand and hangs up on the call. It's 1am and I am calling a client's mobile number! Without a word, I turn and go back to bed.

Whilst my night-time antics can be concerning, the one I cannot believe is my sleep-eating habit. At 3am, Craig shakes me awake. There's a brown mess all over the duvet. Worried that I might have had some kind of problem in the night with my ulcerative colitis, we tear the bed linen from the bed. Hang on, that's not poo: amongst the folds of the duvet cover is a small brown square with a diamond shape on it. Recognising this pattern, we dash down to the dining room. There on the table is all the evidence we need. Strewn across the table, as if attacked by a wild animal, is shredded gold paper and cardboard. What's missing is the Easter egg!

I have absolutely no recollection of eating that Easter egg; there's no taste of it in my mouth, but there's not a shred of chocolate left – just that blob of melted chocolate that made its way back to bed.

Chapter Two

WE'VE BOOKED a holiday to take some time out with the children; since I became poorly, the whole family has been missing out on quality time together, so even though I know this isn't going to be a comfortable journey for me, the holiday is going to be fantastic. We're booked to stay at a Center Parcs holiday village at Eperheide in Belgium, with their indoor play areas, aqua park and all the amazing outdoor space for the children to run wild for a week. We are travelling by car on the ferry. However, another issue that has arisen as a result of being stuck on the toilet for up to an hour each time, multiplied by several times a day, is that I am suffering from piles. When my body goes into spasms from the ulcerative colitis, trying to evacuate what feels like all my internal organs, this involuntary spasming causes a great deal of pressure on the bowel, resulting in the most uncomfortable, and sometimes painful, piles. But we've even thought of a solution for this, and that is a rubber ring. This ring won't be seeing any kind of aqua activity – it's purely going to be my seat for the car journey. I cannot say I am looking forward to the miles and miles of travelling, especially

TWO

looking for emergency pit stops along the way, but we all need to get away.

On Friday afternoon, we drive up from north Devon to Buckinghamshire, where we are staying over at my mum's house before we head down to Dover for the ferry. This gives me a good four-hour practice journey with the ring, which, whilst not the softest of seats, definitely does take the pressure off the piles. At five and three years old, the children are excited about going on a ferry. They've been looking at photographs of the boat, wanting to know how big it is, what it's called and how long we will be on it for. This is a trip of a lifetime for them, and at last I feel like I'm able to give them something to smile about.

Saturday morning, we wake at 4am to prepare for our drive to Dover. The car is still all packed up from yesterday afternoon's drive, so there isn't much to do: just get the children up and dressed, grab a coffee, thank Mum for the overnight accommodation, and then we can be on our way.

'Craig, look at Natasha!'

Aghast, I carry Natasha through to our bedroom. She is covered in red spots. Not just on her face, but down her arms, and they are appearing on her tummy and back as well. The whole house is now awake at this unearthly hour, and we roll a glass over Natasha's arms to check that this isn't meningitis or something awful.

'I think, Caroline, that looks like chicken pox,' says Mum, who's obviously seen me and my sisters go through this many years ago.

'Oh, no! Does that mean we can't go away? Or is it that because she now has the spots she's not contagious, because I recall they're only contagious in the period before the spots come out?'

My head is reeling, trying to remember when a child is classed as contagious, and now worrying that this is going to ruin the holiday. We call the out-of-hours doctors and go through the whole procedure of answering their questions and ask the one question that I dread to know the answer to. Does this mean we cannot take her on the ferry to Belgium?

'I'm sorry, but with her spots you won't be able to take her abroad. Even though she is past the contagious stage, she clearly looks like she's got chicken pox and the holiday park will likely ask that you keep her indoors the whole time so she cannot pass anything on to other children.'

I cannot believe this! We've had the worst few years ever, we book a holiday and now we cannot go. We're all upset, none more so than Robert, who was so looking forward to going on the ferry. I know there's nothing we can do about this, but I feel terrible for him as his little face crumples in tears. We have no option but to go back home.

Back in Devon, we take stock of the situation as Natasha recovers from the chicken pox. Maybe it had been a blessing in disguise that we didn't drive all the way to Belgium with me sitting on a rubber ring. Who knows how I would have fared on the journey. We book something closer to home: a week at Butlins, Minehead. It's not the special holiday we had hoped to give the children, but they are happy to be going away.

Considering this is just an hour from home, the journey with the rubber ring is terribly uncomfortable for me and it's a relief to actually reach our destination. We check in and find our way to our little holiday chalet for the week. The children are excited to be here, with so much to see and do. At last we can be like any other family and relax with all the food and entertainment laid

TWO

on. This should take the stress off me for the week and keep things under control.

The main indoor pavilion area is vast, with a stage that hosts a huge variety of shows and acts for the children, from Bob the Builder to the Skyline Gang. Surrounded by coffee shops, games machines, puppet shows and sweet shops, there's so much to do. Heading to the fairground outside, I feel that awful cramping feeling coming on, doubling me up in pain. The ulcerative colitis is increasingly worsening, and I make a mad dash to the ladies' toilet, yet again leaving Craig hanging around outside with the children. Thankfully there's no queue, but, knowing that I am losing control of my bodily functions, I head for the cubicle in the furthest corner. As my body erupts, I curl up inside at the embarrassment of this horrible disease. No one wants to have their life ruled by toilets and loo roll.

As I hear people coming and going in the other cubicles, I am acutely aware that I've been locked in here for over half an hour. It's not that I have any choice in the matter: my body is just continuously spasming. After an endless time, I re-emerge to find my family kicking their heels, hanging around the games area nearest the toilets. I am feeling wobbly and weak. The blood loss I suffer with these attacks is profuse. For me this is becoming an everyday occurrence – and I know it's the disease, but I feel I am falling apart.

I'm so exhausted, I admit defeat in tears, choosing to go back to the chalet whilst Craig takes the children off to the fairground. I cannot let my children's holiday be spoiled by constantly hanging around toilet doors or spending it cooped up in the chalet with me. The family come back to check on me later in the afternoon; I've been laid up on the bed for the whole afternoon and I ache all over. We head out for dinner in the large dining hall, where the choice of food for me is very limited, as I am still trying to avoid anything that might set off the bloating and trigger another attack. I am becoming fearful of what to eat these days; and, although I just pick at food, the bloating effect of the steroids makes me look obese, and that's depressing me further.

The week continues in the same vein: I make an attempt to go for breakfast and find some activity with the children, only to be rushing back to the chalet at the slightest indication of stomach cramp. I'm spending more and more time each day just stuck indoors, dreading even leaving the chalet. Craig and the children, I know, are missing me being a part of all their enjoyment, and inside I am crying every time they go out and I stay behind. I am trying my best to put a brave face on things, but I'm not coping with it very well at all.

By the end of the week, the children have done everything on the site a hundred times and have had a fantastic time with some freedom to run wild; Craig is very much like a single parent now. I am becoming invisible within my own family and it's heartbreaking.

* * * * *

Work is becoming increasingly difficult to manage. The steroids are seriously messing with my head, and I am finding it difficult to concentrate for any length of time. I'm fortunate to have two members of staff – Sally and Beth – who have been keeping everything ticking over, but I am the one who has to go out and win the new business. Without new clients and projects coming through the doors, the workload is drying up, but I am

TWO

increasingly having to take 'power naps' in the office in the afternoon as the fatigue washes over me.

With my determination not to let this disease beat me, I head out to meet a potential new client to discuss the design of their brochure. Walking through town towards the car park, that ominous cramping starts. I'm on a street with lots of little gift shops and no public toilets anywhere in sight. There is, thankfully, a large pub on the corner, and I make a beeline for it. Being only mid-morning, this less than salubrious pub doesn't yet have any customers in, but the doors are open and I shoot through them like a rocket. As I scan around for the sign for the toilets, I ask the woman behind the bar where the loos are.

'We're not a public convenience, you know,' she grumbles at me.

'I'm sorry, but I have an illness that means I have to go to the toilet urgently.' As I spot the toilet sign at the back of the room, the woman continues to berate me.

'We all have things wrong with us,' she continues to moan. 'We don't allow people to just come in here and use our toilets. We pay water rates and everything, so unless you're a customer, they're not for public use.'

Doubled up holding my stomach, I snap back, 'I'm sorry I don't look sick, but if I stand here any longer, you're going to have a bigger problem on your hands.' With that I run for the toilets, slamming the door and locking myself in just in time.

It's a sorry state when there's such a lack of awareness and understanding of Crohn's and colitis. This debilitating disease is more common than people think, and so often misunderstood as IBS. It's at moments like this that a little compassion would have helped, rather than adding to the anxiety and upset. I've now got to confront the wrath of this woman when I leave and goodness knows when that could be!

Client meetings are now also becoming increasingly difficult. Later the same day I find myself sat in a meeting with a potential new tourist attraction client, discussing the design of their new brochure. Usually I plan meetings at a time when my body typically behaves itself, but today I've got an afternoon appointment. I've tried not to eat, but that seems to be as bad for the bloating as eating is. Sat in a small room, I can feel my stomach beginning to churn. If I can just get through this meeting quickly, I might be OK. I'm fooling myself, of course, and as I feel the need to go to the toilet coming on, I break out in a hot sweat, fearing what might happen. I have no option but to interrupt the meeting suddenly and find their toilets, which are in an outside block. It's embarrassing enough to suddenly dash out of a one-to-one meeting, but then sitting in the loo for a good 20 minutes, I am surprised they didn't send out a search party for me. What must they think? Coming back to the meeting room, the man has been getting on with his work and I apologise profusely. How do you tell a potential new client that you are so ill that you nearly pooed yourself? I didn't actually say this to him, but just made an excuse that I was unwell. It's just so unprofessional! Needless to say, we didn't win the business.

In the office, things are getting tough: the work is drying up and I am seriously having to think about letting one of my two staff go to keep costs down. But who? Beth, the account executive, who works with the clients and does the copywriting, or Sally, the office manager, who takes away all the stress and worry for me on the accounts side? It's a really hard thing to consider. If I lose Beth,

TWO

I will have to deal with the current client workload as well as new business searching, but could my body cope with more meetings? If I lose Sally, I'll have to take on doing the accounts as well as new client searching. But with my head in such a mess, I am struggling to cope. I am completely open and honest with them and put them both on notice of redundancy. I feel awful – it's only a couple of months until Christmas and I've been on the receiving end of redundancy before myself. This disease really sucks.

* * * * *

At home I am spending more and more time in the toilet. The steroid dosage is now at the highest level, and we still cannot get this under control for any length of time. As soon as it seems to be calming, we reduce the tablets and it flares up again. I'm completely washed out by it all. I've become accustomed to taking a magazine or book to the loo with me, as it helps as a distraction from the pain when I'm in there. Some days it can be just too much and overwhelms me. The effect of the tablets, the pained and drained state I'm in, and the sheer depression of having no life or business leaves me in floods of tears in the toilet. Craig has been doing everything around the house – cooking, cleaning, taking care of the kids and taking care of me. Now he sits outside the toilet door and talks to me hour after hour, trying to calm my sobbing. Somehow we have to find a way to overcome this. We've been coping for nearly four years since I was first diagnosed, and we've pulled together to overcome tough times before.

In sheer agony from the piles, I visit my GP, who confirms that they are seriously bad. The way in which these are treated is to have them surgically removed at the hospital. He puts in a call and arranges for me to go to the hospital immediately. Craig, with the children in tow, takes me to the North Devon District Hospital, where I am taken to a ward with other patients. The agony is beyond that of childbirth, and I cannot move for the pain. I cling on to the end of the bed whilst we wait for a doctor to come and see me. The wait seems endless and I cannot help crying from the pain. I feel terrible for my kids to see me like this. Eventually I am seen and told that I will need to stay overnight. Shockingly, I am now told that having the piles surgically removed is 'not how we do it these days'. All I am given is painkillers and ice. *Ice*! I spend the next 24 hours laid up in a hospital bed, with patients shrieking through the night, with an ice pack on my bum! Not wanting to spend another sleepless night in that ward, I am discharged with a large box of rubber gloves.

Those rubber gloves are my saving grace, filled with water and put in the freezer. I can only leave it to the imagination to consider how a frozen finger would rest between my butt cheeks in order to totally numb the area. This and painkillers get me through the coming weeks, but I have now become completely housebound. Not only did I have to let Sally go at the office, but also Beth has now resigned as she can see that we are struggling. Just as I thought I could muddle through with one person, I am left with no one. All I can do is keep the client accounts that I still have ticking over – thankfully they are up country and are accustomed to everything being done via email and telephone, so they have no idea what I am going through. All I have to do is keep things moving from my bed.

My blood counts are really poor and I am constantly fatigued, and now we cannot get this bad flare-up under

TWO

control. My GP and hospital consultant are concerned, and I am admitted to hospital for a course of intravenous steroids. I am now having to consider the possibility that I might need to have major surgery to have my colon and intestines removed, but my heart and head do not want to accept this happening; I've always pushed this to the back of my mind.

With my private medical insurance, I am given a room to myself at North Devon District Hospital. I need to be hooked up to a drip to have steroids fed into my body every six hours – not just for a day, but for a whole week! No going home, no doing any work, no putting Robert and Natasha to bed every night. I've become the invisible mum at home, and now I've been tucked away in a private ward in hospital, being woken through the night as well, for my intravenous steroids. To boot, my consultant has said I need to have a blood transfusion. I've never wanted a blood transfusion; the thought terrifies me. The consultant puts the facts to me about it and, to be honest, my body is in no fit state to make up the red blood cells itself – it's battling the disease. So I concede that this is an inevitability, and the transfusion is planned to take place whilst I am here in the hospital.

This small magnolia-coloured cell couldn't be more boring. Four plain walls are all I have to stare at for a week. The only exception is the TV monitor that swivels from the wall behind me, with a limited choice of rubbish programmes to watch. I've a stack of magazines and puzzle books to try to fill the hours between nurse visits, when they take blood samples, check my blood pressure and plug the steroid injection into the cannula, a thin tube, that's been inserted into the vein on the back of my left hand. Another machine is wheeled into the room to administer the blood transfusion. This isn't going to be a quick thing, and as they put another cannula into my right arm, I settle myself down for another long, boring day, but this time with no mobility for a few hours.

As the transfusion comes to an end, a strange sensation comes over me. It's like waking up from a groggy sleep. As the hours slip by I'm feeling brighter, more refreshed. In fact, I feel like I've been on a night out – my body is buzzing. Having healthy blood pumping through my veins, I cannot believe how alive I feel. When Craig and the children come to visit me, they can see a distinct change in me. Whilst I would never have wanted a blood transfusion, I confess that it was absolutely the right thing to do, but I wasn't to know that until after feeling the effects.

A couple of weeks later, I'm heading out for that fateful cinema trip with Craig, when it all starts to unravel again, and tough choices have to be made.

'You are the only one who can make this decision. It will have an impact on all of us, but it's in your hands. I'll support you whatever you choose, but it's time for you to choose.' The words of my husband are rolling around in my head, words I knew I'd have to hear but never really wanted to hear spoken out loud; it made it all so real. I've got to make the biggest decision of my life: a decision I could never have imagined having to make. Major surgery looms, and I am facing the unknown.

Sat on the comfy old brown sofa in our lounge, it's as though the walls are listening. This Victorian house, with its high ceilings and traditional fireplace, must have witnessed so many events over the decades, but I wonder if it's ever seen this? The kids are safely tucked up in bed, not knowing the drama that is playing out just a floor below.

TWO

To them, this is just your regular old Saturday night; to me, it's a turning point. I can see in his eyes that Craig's words are sincere; my eyes are wet with emotion. This is so bloody awful!

Chapter Three

WEARING THE familiar blue hospital gown, tied loosely at the back, I walk nervously towards the pre-op room at the BUPA hospital next door to Frenchay Hospital, Bristol.

This morning I had woken in familiar surroundings, staying at my sister-in-law's house last night with my family around me. Now they have dropped me off at the hospital, knowing that today is the day that my surgery is going to take place: 20 March 2009. The hospital is more like a smart hotel, which takes away some of the clinical fear that is growing inside me. I've a private room with a large en-suite shower room. If it wasn't for all the technology hooked up along the wall, it really could pass as a decent hotel room.

After putting all my belongings in the cupboard, Craig, Robert, Natasha and I go for a wander outside in the sunshine. Whilst I'm in here today, Craig is taking the children to Bristol Zoo, but we have explained to them that being here is going to make Mummy well. At just six and four years old, they've no conception of what's really happening, but they know they've got a day trip out of

THREE

it. After a final hug, they head off as I turn back into the building where my life is about to change forever.

As the nurse walks with me into the pre-op room, I feel my legs are wobbly at the thought of what is about to happen. I had a second blood transfusion just a few days ago at my local hospital, to ensure that my body was suitably 'topped up' with good red blood cells to be able to heal from surgery. At the same time, the stoma care nurse and I had discussed where my stoma was to be positioned on my body and marked it with a black 'X' in permanent marker. A stoma is formed from the end of the intestine, which is brought through an incision in the abdominal wall, so the body's waste will go into a stoma bag, as a result of my large intestine, colon and rectum being removed. It's bizarre what influences your decisions. My biggest concern was whether I'd be able to wear hipster jeans. Resigning myself to the fact that there are only so many options for the site of my stoma, I guess the jeans from now on will most likely be high waisted.

Apart from Natasha's birth, I have never had surgery and I've definitely never been anaesthetised. As I lie down on the trolley, the surgeon I met earlier in the day, who discussed the whole procedure with me, gives me a reassuring smile and introduces me to the anaesthetist, who's going to be monitoring me throughout. It's all feeling a little surreal; panic is rising; why do I have to be here, so alone; I don't like this; I'm scared. Tears start to run down my face – I am absolutely terrified that I will never wake up again and see my kids. This could be the end, and the last people I will see are these strangers all scrubbed up for surgery.

Seeing how upset I am, and that I am trying so desperately to hold it together, the nurse takes my hand, talking to me as the anaesthetist inserts the tube into the cannula in my left arm.

'It's all OK, Caroline, the anaesthetist will be looking after you throughout.'

'I'm scared,' I cry.

'I promise you're going to be OK. We are just going to make you go to sleep and it will all be over before you know it. Now count backwards for me from 10.'

'10 … 9 …… 8 …… 7 ………' I lose consciousness.

Later: 'Bleep …… Bleep …… Bleep …… Bleep ……'

I slowly come round to the sound of bleeping beside me. Stirring slowly, I look around the room through heavy eyes. The scenery around me is different. It's a much larger room, with a couple of nurses buzzing around and shuffling papers. In the recovery room, I am the only patient and the nurse quickly comes over to see how I'm doing. I've monitors stuck on my body.

'It's all done,' the nurse says. 'We need you to rest in here whilst you recover from the anaesthetic, then we will take you back to your room in a bit.'

It's the most weird feeling. As I come round more fully, I don't feel like I've been asleep. It feels like someone just turned out the light one moment and flicked it back on the next. There is no sensation of time passing at all.

The surgeon comes to visit me with a great big smile.

'Well, Caroline, you are all sorted now. The operation went well and I can tell you that you are the first person in the world to have this particular surgery performed through single-site keyhole. It took us about an hour longer than it usually would, at three and a half hours.'

Three and a half hours! It feels like no time at all, but now it's early evening. I knew I was going to be having keyhole surgery and expected to have up to five puncture

THREE

wounds through which the cameras and medical devices would be inserted. But in fact this amazing surgeon has just performed the whole surgery through a single keyhole incision. That single keyhole is now where the end of my small intestine comes through my stomach wall and forms my stoma. I have no scars across my abdomen at all. My rectum has been removed and sewn up, and I now have a 'Barbie butt'.

As my ulcerative colitis had been inflamed throughout my colon and large intestine, I'd had to make a really hard choice about my surgery. I could have had the ileostomy and left my rectum in situ, giving me the option, later on, of having a reversal. If I did choose to have my intestines rejoined to my rectum, I would need up to two further surgeries, creating an internal pouch from my small intestine. Even then, there would be no guarantee that this would work, and I could end up with proctitis, which is an inflammation of the lining of the rectum, causing pain and that feeling of urgency to use the toilet. I also had the issue that the ulcerative colitis had been right through my colon from my rectum; leaving the rectum in place, even with my ileostomy, I'd still have the same problems with UC in that area. It was therefore a no-brainer for me. If I wanted my quality of life back, I was going to opt for the full non-reversible option. Why go through all this pain and surgery without some guaranteed life afterwards? Plus it would not mean spending the rest of my life wondering whether or not to have a reversal.

'You won't be needing any of these now,' says the ward doctor, as he packs away all the boxes of tablets and medication that I have come to rely on over these last four years. From taking 16 tablets daily, I am immediately cut to just a couple of steroid tablets per day from now on, and that just needs to be reduced gradually so my body doesn't go into a trauma state from going 'cold turkey'. The feeling of being seriously ill one minute and then being totally cured the next is surreal. Those months and years of suffering are gone in an instant.

When Craig and the children come to visit me a little later, I am beaming from ear to ear. The tears that roll down my face are those of joy; of relief. I feel as though over these recent years I have been continuously tortured, and now it's suddenly stopped. No pain, no urgency: my body is calm and resting. It's going to take a while to mentally adjust to some form of normality. Attached to the right side of my abdomen, below my belly button, hangs an ostomy bag. It's not at all discreet, with its clear front so I can see all the output in the bag. At this stage, I need to be able to see what I'm doing and how I will need to put this on every time it needs a change. I view it like changing a baby's nappy. It's not the most pleasant task, but it's an everyday normal thing to do now, and it's saved my life.

So many people suffer with Crohn's and ulcerative colitis in silence. They've become accustomed to saying they're OK, when really they're not OK. It's like a taboo subject, something to hide away and not admit to suffering with. The excruciating pain, however, can wear you down. Many confront depression as a result and at its worst, some do not survive – choosing to take their own life rather than live with the pain. I didn't know anyone with Crohn's or colitis when I was diagnosed, so I understand what a dark, lonely place that can be.

*****

Within 24 hours in my own hospital room, I've quickly taken to being able to empty my bag and change it myself.

THREE

It only took the stoma nurse one visit to show me how to remove the bag, clean the skin around the stoma and stick a new bag on. I am so determined to get home that I'm not squeamish about it. I've lived with a lot worse for years now, so having this bag makes life so much easier. I am now in control of my body, and that's the best feeling in the world.

With a final visit from the stoma nurse a day later, I am signed off as being suitably able to be 'self-caring'. From surgery on Friday night, I am heading home on Monday, laden with my new parcel of ostomy supplies and instructions to rest for the next six weeks. Whilst there's no scarring on the outside of my body, my internal organs have been thrown about a bit, and the incision through the wall of my abdomen will need to heal internally, just like having the caesarean.

Taking a week of total rest, I'm not allowed to lift a hoover or even a kettle, so poor Craig has to run around after me again and keep the house and family in order. Into the second week, I pick up my laptop, prop up the pillows on my bed and start reconnecting with clients. The first one asks if I've had a nice holiday. Pah! If only he knew. I had consciously not told any clients that I was ill and due to have surgery, for fear that they'd think I couldn't cope and cancel their contracts. I couldn't afford to lose any clients, so I'd kept working from my laptop at home whilst I was ill and had just told them I was off for a week. Being housebound didn't stop me being able to write press releases and articles, or liaise with editors on the phone. With no staff, I'd had to retain as much as I could. Now I could pick up where I'd left off, and start to look at rebuilding our crumbling business from scratch.

I thought that once I'd had the surgery and got my ileostomy bag, my body would be just fine. With the steroids now reduced to a very minimal level since the surgery, surely I would be fit and well to get out there with the children and be a real mum. When I wake up one morning, however, and find that I cannot easily walk down the stairs, I think I've made a bad decision. The knuckles in my hands have been stiffening up recently, but now my hips and knees are going too. I physically cannot walk down the stairs. In a three-storey Victorian town house, there are a lot of stairs, and I have to resort to holding the banister and side-stepping my way up and down them. Clearly, this is the impact of having been on some nasty medication for so long and now my body is rebelling. The only thing I can do is keep moving; I have to try to loosen up all my joints and endeavour to get my mobility back. It takes a couple of weeks for the knees and hips to get easier, after I'm sent to a specialist who recommended that I continue to take calcium tablets. He wants to keep an eye on what looked like the onset of osteoarthritis, which is the side effect of the steroids. I'm in my early 40s and I am moving like someone in their 90s. Having fought so hard to get my quality of life back to enjoy with my family, I cannot let something else stop me. I am going to have to make sure I regularly do the exercises I have been given to keep the joints flexible.

I've never been a particularly sporty person; to be honest, I've been a couch potato all my life. At high school I would walk around the cross-country running course, and in hockey I made sure I was always picked as the goalkeeper, as I found running made me very breathless. I'd had a couple of asthma attacks when I was younger, and I guess I'd come to use this as an excuse not to do any

THREE

running about. I didn't like running, and I was terrified of water after an incident as a young child when I was dunked unexpectedly and had a panic attack. Ever since, I have had an inherent fear of drowning, so I never go swimming. In a pool or on a beach, I always stay well inside the shallow area.

So now I am confronted with having to do more exercise to keep my mobility. Looking in the mirror, all I can see is this very bloated, overweight individual who's now got no guts and has to wear a bag hanging from her tummy for the rest of her life. The bag is my saviour for my health and my family, but now I need to take some time to get myself back to being me.

Nine months after surgery, I decide that the only way I am going to make myself do any kind of regular exercise is to set myself a target. I simply don't have the motivation to go out every day for a short run: there has to be a purpose, a reason to go out. Scanning the internet, I come across a charitable event that involves cycling. Now, cycling I can do! I had taken part in a cycle event ten years prior to my illness, cycling 400km in six days through the Rift Valley in Kenya on a mountain bike, in aid of Scope. There is actually a possibility that that trip had been a trigger for my ulcerative colitis, as I had succumbed to giardiasis on that trip – a form of dysentery – and it was suggested that the parasite had remained dormant in the gut. But who knows? There is currently no confirmed evidence, to my knowledge, that this is what caused my immune disorder.

This cycle event, though, really appeals to me; cycling is easier than my loathed running. I need a challenge, and this event could well be that challenge for me. It is again raising money for Scope, but it is cycling from London to

Paris in 24 hours in the coming July. Considering it is now November, that doesn't give me very long, but I could get a friend to join me and we can do it as a relay team.

'You are mad, Caroline,' says one of my oldest friends, Doreen Gowing, who is a keen cyclist and someone I know who would be able to take on an epic cycle ride and would be a fantastic team-mate.

'Do you realise how far London to Paris is? And do you realise the speed you will need to average to achieve this?' Doreen throws all sorts of questions at me, but I've got my heart set on this goal. Despite having had major surgery earlier this year, I am excited at the prospect of being out on the road, having my freedom back, and being able to not only get myself fit, but prove to myself and to others that having an ileostomy has been a good decision and to live life to the max.

Doreen would be the first to admit that my enthusiasm for the event, together with my self-assured belief that we can do this and get to Paris in 24 hours, is what convinced her to sign up with me. Now all I have to do is start cycling to get in some practice, and get fundraising. But first of all, I need to have a conversation with my GP about this, to see if there are any reasons why I might not be able to take on such a mammoth event.

'Don't expect too much of your body, Caroline,' said my GP, with a pitying look on her face. 'You've had major surgery and you've got an ileostomy now. Your body is not like it was before.'

Waves of devastation and disappointment are mingled with a bloody-mindedness. OK, so I am struggling with osteoarthritis-like symptoms, but at least I can now get outside and be active. I assure her that the exercise and movement have definitely been helping with the stiffness

THREE

in my joints. With pleading eyes, I check with her that there would be no harm in at least giving this a go.

'See how you get on with the exercises and training then, but I wouldn't commit to being able to do the event,' she says with a weak smile. I am sure in her head she's thinking, 'poor lady so wants to try; she's been through so much, might as well let her.' In my head I am hearing, 'OK, so that's a go!' loud and clear.

Chapter Four

WITHIN THE next two months, I go for my check-up with the consultant about the osteoarthritis-type symptoms. I skip through the door to his surgery, smiling. I cannot wait to tell him what I've got planned. Added to this, I cannot wait to tell him that all the stiff joints and arthritic pain have gone – totally gone! The regular exercise has completely eradicated the pains I was having. He's stunned when I show him the range of movement in my joints – it's quite miraculous. He's buoyed by my announcement about riding London to Paris in 24 hours, but finishes the consultation with a wary little 'Let's see how you're doing in six months' time.' Well, six months later I had to cancel my appointment with him: there was no point – I was totally mobile and pain-free.

Signing up for London to Paris in 24 hours was maybe slightly foolhardy, but I need a goal to aim for. I need to exercise, and now I have a purpose. I seek out a personal trainer who can help. Neil Harris comes recommended, and he's local. We have one of those pre-training discussions where you take all your measurements and weight; we discuss previous fitness (in my case, almost

FOUR

zero) and what you want to achieve – er … cycle London to Paris in 24 hours, and we've only got seven months until the event. I am starting to become accustomed to the look of shock on people's faces when I say this. Yes, I know it's a tall order, but I've got a ton of determination. I tell Neil that in order to achieve this within 24 hours, the information pack says you need to be averaging a cycle speed of 18mph.

'Don't you mean 18km per hour?' he asks. '18mph is a pretty fast average over 270 miles, and we're starting from scratch.'

I show him the information pack and he sits back. 'OK, so we've got a lot of work to do!'

Training starts in earnest. Neil really has got a task on his hands to get me anywhere near fit enough to get this average speed, so it's back to basics. Whilst I thought we would immediately jump on to our bikes and go out cycling, I couldn't be more wrong. He has a tough regime of circuit training lined up for me, to start getting back in shape. Before I am even ready for my Barbie butt to touch my saddle, I am going to have to build up my core strength, lose some of this blubber and build up some cardiovascular endurance.

As he turns up for our first training session at my house, he's come prepared with every form of 'torture' an unfit person like me could imagine. There are dumb-bells and a balance ball, elastic straps, floor ladders, an exercise mat and so much more. Even the warm-up of floor exercises is tough for my stiff old body. At home I have a dusty old cross-trainer from back in the days when I had my first child, Robert – I used to use it every morning to lose weight after he was born. Now it has gathered dust for many years. No longer will it be confined to the corner as a coat stand: it's wheeled out and Neil cranks up the gearing on it so I'm getting some good resistance. After an hour, I feel like I've been through the wringer but I am buzzing. Neil leaves me with an exercise regime to carry out regularly throughout the week until our next training session.

Starting to train in the winter is not the most sensible idea. As my indoor circuit training is paying dividends, it's time to get out on the bike. However, with the weather so wet and cold, Neil insists I join him on my mountain bike. This hasn't had a saddle on it for ten years, since my charity ride through Kenya, so the bike gets treated to a service and I have to 'man up' and brave the weather. It's time for my big pink bike to do what it was designed to do. After loading it on to the car, I drive over to the meet point to join Neil at Braunton. We are going to start building some power into my legs and are going for a 14-mile ride along the Tarka Trail to Barnstaple.

Never have I hated a ride more than on this day. The sun is up and I am wrapped up warm, but I had not appreciated the wind-chill factor on my hands. All we are doing is a flat ride, but my hands are numb from the cold. My breathing is laboured at the intensity of being out on the bike, and I could cry. 'What on earth am I trying to prove? I hate this – why did I have to be so stupid as to sign up for this event? I am never going to make it.' The realisation of exactly how hard this is going to be is dawning on me, as Neil rides ahead, shouting back over his shoulder, 'You have got to catch me.' This fartlek training (bursts of speed, then steady slower sections) is absolutely exhausting. But, like a greyhound being released from the blocks as the hare shoots by, my competitive streak kicks in. I have to catch him. No matter what he does, I cannot

FOUR

back down. I am going to get on to his back wheel. And I do.

Our weekly rides get longer and longer. If I thought riding along the flat Tarka Trail was tough, I'm in for a whole new level of pain when he leads me off down to a beach – a pebble beach. From a fartlek session between speed humps in the road, heading out to Crow Point, Neil turns off and takes us down on to the deserted beach. Trying to ride across slippery pebbles is an art form. My back wheel slips this way and that as Neil dashes ahead of me. Flicking sea-polished stones left, right and centre, it's a blessing to reach the damp sand. Or is it? The weight of the sand clogs up the grip on my tyres, and I can feel the difference in both the weight of the bike and the handling. This is a tougher workout than I had imagined. Being a cold wintry morning, the pathways off the beach are deserted and we skirt around frozen puddles. My hands and face are burning from the cold, but as we get back to the car I feel more alive than I have done for many years.

As the months slip by and spring approaches, I can see and feel the difference in my legs; my quads are beefing up and I am feeling powerful out on the mountain bike. Now it's time to take it up a notch and take my road bike out. As we head out, Neil still on his mountain bike and me on my old Peugeot Audax, I can feel the tarmac slipping away under my wheels so much quicker. With slick tyres on my road bike, the power I have built up in my legs comes into its own. It's like jumping from an old, worn-out bike to a rocket-fuelled one. Our weekly rides are not only getting longer, but they are also getting more hilly. There's no point just being able to ride on the flat: I am going to have to be able to take on some hills. Our long Saturday ride each week becomes an adventure, and I start to take on ascents that I'd previously seen as my nemesis. Living in Ilfracombe, every direction starts with a hill climb, and this morning Neil has planned to start the ride from here. We begin with a steady two-mile climb and enjoy riding out in the late spring sunshine towards Exmoor. From the top of Ilfracombe, the roads are undulating with stunning views, so we enjoy some fantastic routes that lead us down towards Lynton and Lynmouth, an iconic location with two villages that are joined by a water-powered funicular railway. The descent towards Lynton is long and winding, but, for every amazing downhill ride, there's going to be a killer climb on the other side.

We find ourselves heading down into the Valley of the Rocks, with its stunning lunar rock formations covered in wild goats. This is one of the most beautiful local areas to visit, but I can see the size of the climb on the opposite side of the valley, with its switchbacks. I blanch at the thought of what is about to come; I grit my teeth and dig deep, ready for a long, hard climb. 'My legs are pistons, my legs are pistons,' I repeat over and over to myself as I get higher and higher.

Whilst Neil zips up the hill as light-footed as one of the wild goats, I grind out the gears at a slower but steady pace. It wasn't that long ago when I couldn't even get up out of my saddle and on to my pedals – my legs just hadn't been strong enough – but now I hop in and out of the saddle to make it all the way to the top. Looking back down to where we have come from, I cannot believe I have made it.

* * * * *

'My legs are pistons, my legs are pistons.' This has become my mantra when I tackle any hill. I can envisage my legs pumping up and down just like the pistons under

FOUR

the bonnet of a supercar. It is Doreen who has got me visualising myself powering up these hills. She has created for me a hypnotherapy recording, so that I can focus on my own self-belief. It is her voice that rings in my head, reminding me that my legs are pistons.

All those years ago, before I had gone out on the charity ride to Kenya, I had signed up to ride through the Grand Canyon, but disaster had struck on a regular Sunday morning bike ride with Doreen. Heading out from my family home in Beaconsfield, Bucks, we had only been out on the road for about a mile. Before the days of having any really serious cycling gear, I was wearing only a pair of shorts and a sporty little crop top, as it was a hot day, plus of course the compulsory crash helmet. There are some fabulous hills around the area, and as we came to the top of a particularly exciting descent, Doreen mentioned that our friend Denise Parker had clocked 40mph on a downhill. This sounded exciting, so I had no qualms at all about giving this hill everything I'd got. Pedalling hard as I started the descent, I quickly picked up speed. With one eye on the CatEye speedometer that I had on my handlebars, I was determined to hit that 40mph.

Coming towards the bottom of the hill, having hit my top speed, it all went wrong. I knew these roads well and knew that there would soon be a sharp left turn at the bottom, so I started to brake. The road curved slightly to the right, but at speed my left pedal caught the edge of the kerb. It was too late to react, and I was catapulted off my bike on to the pathway. I slid on my left side along the ground, followed rapidly by my bike. I came to a halt as I hit a grassy verge with tall poplar trees surrounding the front garden of a very expensive house. Afraid I might have broken something, I lay still as Doreen dashed to my side. The owners of the house happened to arrive from down the road and drove around me to get into their driveway. No stopping, no coming back out to check I was OK.

I'd not broken anything, but I had totally lacerated the left side of my body. My ankle, knee, hip and left arm were all bleeding. My crop top was no longer covering the parts of my body that it ought to have been covering; my left nipple was exposed and bleeding. An old man driving a car pulled up, seeing my crumpled body on the grass verge. His kind offer of assistance was gratefully received, but, up on my feet, I wasn't going to need an ambulance (though I kept my hand over my left breast for the sake of decency). I must have been a sight for sore eyes as another car pulled up to help. This time it was someone I knew, and she was a district nurse. Her deft hands set to work cleaning up my wounds as best she could on the roadside, sufficient for me to be able to get back on my bike. I had no way of getting back to my house without riding; after pushing my bike, which had only received a bent brake handle and a few scuffs on the pedal, back up the hill, the adrenaline rush kept the pain at bay and we cycled home.

* * * * *

It's a misty 6am start in a hotel in London on a Friday morning. Never have I seen so much Lycra in one place. The room is full of almost 140 eager cyclists, from novices to those thinking they are as good or as fast as the professionals. There's a tangible excitement in the air as we all fill our water bottles and collect our bikes from the storage area, which in fact is the hotel's main conference room. My bike preparation routine entails some extra

FOUR

baggage – packing my emergency stoma supplies in a saddlebag. We won't have access to our rucksacks until we get to the feed stations, and our cases won't be seen until we get to Paris. So I need to be thoroughly prepared throughout this journey.

Blackheath in London is the start of this inaugural event organised by Scope, the charity for those with a disability. The queues for the toilets are endless, but gradually everyone wheels their trusty steeds out on to the open green expanse of Blackheath, where there's racking for the bikes and a huge inflatable start-line gantry. Fences on either side funnel us like sheep heading for a sheep dip. With so many people around, I don't want to lose sight of Doreen, and we stay close to one another alongside some equally nervous-looking ladies. One of them, Lucie Gallen, sidles up beside us as we all listen to the announcements on the tannoy about how epic this event is going to be. We have 24 hours to get to Paris, starting very shortly at 9am. The countdown begins to yelps and cheers, and the ringing of bicycle bells. At last the loud blast of the air-horn releases us and we roll out in convoy under the gantry and on to the roads of London.

As we head out of town up Shooters Hill, the commuters probably hate us. Like a snake we make our way around buses that have pulled in to pick up passengers, whilst cars and vans try to overtake the stream of riders. The faster riders have gone to the front, and little gaps appear between the groups. Ahead we see there's already been a fracas with one of our cyclists and a car, when the vehicle had cut across in front of the bike, to turn left into a driveway, leaving the cyclist nowhere to go but into the side of the car. Getting out of London is clearly going to be a very nerve-racking ride. There are organised feed stations along the route to Paris at various sports halls and school grounds. At the first feed station, after nearly three hours of cycling, those of us who are relaying across the route have to leave one of our team to get on the bus, whilst the other rider continues for a second stint.

Having looked at the route in advance, it was agreed that I would be rider one and do the double stint in the UK, and Doreen would end up having the double stint at the end as we all roll into Paris together. Heading out through the Kent countryside, I am regretting doing the double stint in the UK, as the roads in some places are really quite pot-holed and there are a lot more hills in Kent than I had realised. If I'd thought this was going to be a generally flat ride, I was in for a big shock.

The roads are endless, but I can still see other riders ahead and behind me – so I don't feel deserted, which was my biggest fear. There is a reassurance that we are all in this together and have to just keep slogging on. One hill rolls into the next, and by the time I get to the second feed station I am ready to sit down and rest. The bonus of doing all this cycling is that the feed stations are full of bananas, flapjacks, cake, pasta, nuts, chocolate and sweets. For the first couple of feed station stops, we only get a 15-minute break, such is the pace we have to be setting to get to Paris by tomorrow morning. However, before I can dive into the array of goodies, I have to make a dash to the toilets to sort out my stoma bag. Having an ileostomy means that I have no control over the activity of my output. Where others can just pop to the loo when they feel like it, my ileostomy is constantly working; so, as I get to the feed stations, my bag is filling up and I need to sort this too. The three-hour stints between feed stations is sufficient time for me not to be concerned about stoma bag issues. If

FOUR

I had to go a lot longer without a break, then I could have a problem on the roadside.

Doreen takes the next leg of the ride, which will take us closer to Dover, whilst the bike and I are transported by coach to the next feed station, which is just a few miles outside the Dover ferry port. The pockets of my cycle jersey are stuffed full with energy gels and snack bars; as I drop them into my lap to sit down on the coach, the guy next to me laughs at how much I'm carrying. I am so new to this, I don't really know how much I will need to eat whilst I am actually cycling, so I have come loaded with far too much stuff. Better safe than sorry, is my thinking.

At the next feed station, whilst waiting for Doreen to arrive, I give a live interview with BBC Radio Devon, who have been following my story. Lucie, who I met at the start line, joins me whilst we wait for our team-mates to arrive. The weather is thankfully still dry, albeit starting to become overcast, and the ambience of 70 cyclists who have just ridden from London is electric. There's chat about the roads, the dodgy bits and the great countryside we've ridden through, and more about what is to come. The pressure builds as the riders straggle in; we are all booked on to a ferry at 4pm, so we will have to leave this location in good time to get through customs. Every time a cyclist is spotted coming into the grounds of the school where we are waiting, a cheer goes up; I'm still scanning to see Doreen. Eventually she's in, grinning from ear to ear, with tales from her own 45-mile leg.

Riding into Dover feels like a carnival. Every single rider has regrouped as we are riding in en masse. The organisers release us in large groups, so as not to completely clog up the local road network. We are only five miles from the ferry port.

With our passports in our back pockets, we are filtered through the drive-through terminal to customs control. Two customs officers sit bemused in their little cabin at the barrier, as more and more cyclists pile into this covered area. The weather is turning and it begins to rain, so we are all trying to get in out of the downpour. They are unable to check every single individual passport, and the organisers have made arrangements for us to go through. This covered area is like a massive warehouse, open at both ends. Looking ahead, we can see the ferries; and, like the spread of a contagious disease, the pinging of one cycle bell becomes a cacophony of 140 bells reverberating through the building. Perhaps this is why we were quickly released through the barriers to be on our way?

We roll out on to the wide expanse of tarmac, to be held before the ferry is ready for us. Being such a large group, we are being treated like a lorry – we queue up in the parking bay with vehicles to our left and right, also waiting to board the ferry. Who knows what those travellers must have thought when seeing all these Lycra-clad cyclists sitting on their bikes in the rain, laughing and joking. We are eventually released to board the ferry before the cars and vans. There's no racking for the bikes on the boat, so we are instructed to line them all up against the walls of the car level, sometimes two or three deep. Let's just hope none of them fall over – the effect could be like a pack of dominoes going down.

The ferry crossing will be around 90 minutes, and this will be our only long rest before we finish in Paris. We've formed groups of friends along the way, and we all find seats where we can grab a hot coffee and eat, as well as try to close our eyes. Whilst we are tired from the mileage we

FOUR

have already ridden, 4pm is not a time when your body wants to sleep. Even with our eyes closed, our bodies are on alert and we hear everything that's going on around us. All in all, we don't get much rest.

Reaching the French coastline, we're all down on the car decks with our bikes, waiting for all the cars and vans to leave before we can manoeuvre our way off. There's a triumphant feel in our hearts as we we clip into our pedals and ride off the ferry, down the ramp into France at the port of Calais.

As we leave the industrial-looking port area, the scenery changes to the countryside we were hoping for, which lifts our spirits ready for the next stage. The early-evening riding is enjoyable; the roads are flatter and better maintained, and we are all making good progress. So far I've not had any issues with my stoma bag; I've not had to change it at all. As we leave the evening feed station in the dark, I am one of the backmarkers, and a few miles down the road I can feel the acid burn on my skin around my stoma where the output is getting underneath the base plate; the bag is coming unstuck. I kick myself for not having taken the opportunity to change my bag at that last feed station, whether it had needed it or not. Now I am out in the dark with a problem. I've got my emergency kit with me, but there are no facilities as we are riding into the outskirts of a village.

Being one of the last to leave the feed station, I've buddied up with another lady, Hannah, who seems to be as nervous as me about this event; she's on a hybrid and doesn't have clip-in shoes. I pull over and explain I have a problem. Until now I have told no one on this trip (apart from the organisers) that I have an ileostomy, yet here I now am in the dark, in France, having to tell a total stranger that I have to change my bag in public. I feel embarrassed, but I have no option but to disappear behind a stone wall with the village name etched on it, welcoming people to their village. With a head torch on, I do what I need to and clean myself up. I've learned my lesson: I must change my bag at every feed station whether it needs changing or not, to ensure the adhesion on my skin doesn't cause a problem like this again.

We eventually ride into the next feed station; almost every other rider has been through and gone again. Doreen has been waiting nervously for me; she's not able to go until I am in, and she's been worrying that something has happened. Now I am in she's ready to go, and I wave her farewell until the next stop, which will be in the very early hours of the morning.

My next leg of the ride is from 3am. The feed station transition in the night is longer, giving us a 45-minute break. They have laid on full-blown meals, with hot pasta, meats, cheese and more cake – perfect fuel for us all, as we are flagging from the lack of sleep. This has to be the toughest part of the ride. I'm running on adrenaline, energy bars, chocolate and jelly babies. We are riding through what would be stunning scenery if it were daylight. We cruise through tiny villages in the dark, where all you can hear is the sound of a dog barking after being disturbed by the whirring of wheels going by. The villages are like ghost towns; there is a mysterious feeling about cycling through here, knowing all these people are asleep in their beds whilst we keep on pedalling.

In the open countryside, a thick fog descends. The cold and damp seeps through our clothes and our skin. There's no light pollution out here; all we can see is the white spot on the ground in front of us from our headlights and head

FOUR

torches. My bike has red lights on the spokes, so I look like I'm riding some futuristic bike from the film *Tron*! Whilst everyone laughs jovially about how visible I am from a distance, I know I will be seen by vehicles too. How would they miss me? The early-morning lorries hurtle past us through the fog, which is nerve-racking. They get so close you can feel the rush of air sucking at you as they go by.

The fog is playing tricks on my mind, and the lack of sleep is probably doing so too. The road ahead looks like it's going uphill, but my legs are spinning out faster and faster, so I must be going downhill. It's the most surreal experience. The fog is so deep and the night is so dark, you cannot actually see the road further ahead; my focus is just on that one spot of light a couple of feet ahead.

By 5am I am struggling. We have been fighting our way up a never-ending hill but cannot see the top due to the fog. One of the support vehicles has been driving behind us to protect us on the narrow roads, and as the climb increases my legs slow and come to a halt. I've got nothing left. Hannah and I admit that we are both in difficulty, and, having the support vehicle, we contemplate whether we ought to consider giving up and getting the sweeper van to come and collect us. We need to be at the next feed station for our partners to be released for the final stage before we get to Paris. Not only am I letting myself down, I am letting Doreen down too. Why did I ever think I could do this?

The guys in the support vehicle are experienced cyclists who have done this before, and they know how we're feeling. They make sure we eat some more food and take a gel, and that we've plenty of fluid on the bike. After a hug and a pep talk, we're back on our bikes. As the gel hits my muscles, I find a second wind and keep on pushing. The terrain levels out, and as the fog lifts as the sun rises, I look across the fields of crops and hear the crow of a cockerel. I can do this, I can do this! The support team have called ahead, and Doreen has been released to start her final leg even before I'm in.

As I'm one of the final riders to come in, the coach quickly departs for its next destination, which doesn't give me time for a toilet stop. I'm going to have to sort myself out when we get dropped off, before our final section into Paris.

In the outskirts of Paris, the whole contingent of 140 cyclists reconvene as one group. This is our final stage. The sun is coming up to give us a beautiful morning, and we hear the buzz of a city waking up. As we get closer and closer to the heart of the city, we contend with the influx of vehicles and traffic lights. It's a climb up into the centre as we head towards the Arc de Triomphe. This will be a challenging roundabout like no other! We have a group rider with us to help us round; thankfully it's not as busy as I had expected, but it is still daunting to go three-quarters of the way around the Arc de Triomphe with cars coming at you from every direction. We peel off, and before us lies the Champs Elysees … we are so close. The street has barriers on either side – not for us, but for the Tour de France that is finishing here tomorrow.

Riding down the Champs Elysees, the knack is to get up a bit of speed, because it seems to flatten out the cobbles. This iconic cobbled street has my body reverberating, from my wrists to my eyeballs. One last right turn at the bottom and I am heading towards the finish line in front of the Eiffel Tower. As the countdown clock above the finish line ticks down second by second, I cross the line with seven minutes still to go before the

FOUR

24 hours is up. Shrieks and tears are the celebration, with hugs from Doreen, Lucie, Hannah and all the other riders I have come to know as friends in this epic 24 hours. I have proved to myself that this ileostomy has given me back my life, and I am going to make the most of it. Watching Mark Cavendish and the Tour de France racing in the next morning is the icing on the cake.

Chapter Five

MY CYCLING ambitions from here are sporadic, and that's a generous description. To be honest, I find it far too easy to slip back into my couch potato days. Daily life kicks in as I struggle to rebuild my business. We can no longer support other members of staff, so any work I can win I am doing myself. It's more manageable but no less stressful, being the one to not only bring in PR work for myself, but also graphic design work for Craig. We work well as a team, but equally we suffer as a team when things go sour.

I am also learning how to live with my stoma: I've not found it difficult on a day-to-day basis, as it's become routine, but I am being careful about what I eat. There's a lot that new ostomates are told to avoid due to the risk of a blockage.

Maybe we focus on this so much that we become over-cautious when it comes to food. I've started to eat more and more in my regular diet, but some days it can all go pear-shaped for no apparent reason. For me it can be a combination of something I've eaten and also the stress and anxiety of work.

FIVE

I've spent the day on my own, visiting an exhibition at Olympia, London, grabbing food 'on the hoof'. After eating an appetising-looking hot dog, I am leaving the venue feeling just a little bit off. Nothing to worry about – we all get this feeling after eating sometimes, and I make my way down on to the Underground. I probably should have taken more notice of the queasiness. Packed into a crowded Tube train, I break out into a sweat, the feeling of sickness getting stronger and stronger. I know this feeling: I've experienced it once before when I was trying to get home from a meeting on the motorway and I kept having to pull over on to the hard shoulder to be sick nearly 20 times. When this happens, my stoma goes into overdrive too, and my bag keeps filling with fluid.

Now, on the Underground, I know this is about to happen again. I cannot be sick here in this carriage; once my body starts, it won't stop. As the train pulls into the next station, I dash out of the carriage and up the escalators, feeling dizzy and panic-stricken. At the barrier, I spot a guard and ask where the toilets are.

'Sorry, love, there are no public toilets at this station.'

'I need a toilet right now,' I plead, 'I have a medical condition; something I've eaten has affected me and I urgently need a toilet. It might be food poisoning. I'm going to be really sick.'

I must be as white as a ghost, as he takes pity on me and takes me back to the control room, where a small group of Underground staff are watching all the trains and escalators on their screens. 'Have you been taking anything?' he asks; I must have looked like a wretched soul. I cannot believe I could be thought of like this.

He shows me to the single little toilet, where I drop to my knees and vomit into the toilet bowl. The retching is endless, whilst at the same time my stoma bag fills instantly with fluid. Between bouts of being sick, I have to empty my bag down the toilet, then I'm back down on my knees on the cold floor whilst I am sick yet again. Numerous times a member of staff knocks on the door to check if I'm OK. Initially I say, 'Yes, thanks, I'll be OK,' but as the time slips by and I've been in the toilet for over half an hour, I am aware that I am causing them a problem. The next knock on the door, I open it a little to speak to the kindly woman. This time, she asks if I need medical assistance.

'Yes, I think I do.' I admit defeat in tears. I am in a Tube station somewhere in south London (goodness knows where I am), my body has turned itself inside out, I am now too weak and wobbly to stand and I still have to somehow get home to my mum's place out in Buckinghamshire by train. I'm never going to make it. As I shut myself back in the toilet for my body to convulse again, they ring for an ambulance.

The two paramedics who come to collect me couldn't have been nicer. As they help me to walk to the ambulance, I feel like the general public are all staring. The ambulance is parked on the double yellow lines outside the station, with traffic struggling to go around it. Once on board, one of the paramedics takes down all my details and we talk through what's happened. Despite there being absolutely nothing left inside by body, I still keep convulsing, holding the cardboard bowl 'just in case'.

They give me something to stop the sickness spasms as we hurtle across London. I explain where I am meant to be getting to this afternoon; the paramedic grins and says, 'In that case, let's save you having to traipse through London later; we'll take you to a north London hospital so

FIVE

you won't have far to get home and can get a taxi.' I could have hugged him!

In the early-evening rush hour, the journey is slow and they cheekily tell me they're going to put the 'blues and twos' on to get through quicker. I've never been in an ambulance before, so this is turning into quite an experience. At the hospital, I am taken in on a wheelchair. I could have walked, but I've become so weak and dehydrated they don't want to take the chance of me passing out. Once I am safely put into a room with nurse care, they wish me well and leave. I'm exhausted, and the nurse immediately has me laid out on a bed with an intravenous drip attached to my arm to get me hydrated again. It's now mid-evening, and I am worried about getting back. After a couple of hours attached to the drip, I convince the nurse that I feel well enough to discharge myself. I cannot possibly stay here overnight – I don't even know where 'here' is. At 10.30pm, I hail a taxi and get driven out to Buckinghamshire. That is an experience I never want again. I don't want to feel I cannot go anywhere for fear of a blockage or something upsetting my stomach. It will take some time to feel confident again. After feeling as though life was pretty much back to normal, my body reminds me that I'm not the same as I was.

*****

Two years slip by before my mind is brought back to getting back in the saddle (I said my training was sporadic). This time, it's another organised 24-hour charity ride, but just in the UK. Lucie Gallen and I have remained firm friends after London to Paris, and we've signed up for Newcastle to London 24, alongside Gethin Pearson and James Baggott, both of whom we met on London to Paris.

This time it's a much easier start, heading up together on a train to Newcastle. Our friends and family will be waiting for us in London.

The fact that I've not consistently trained over the last two years means that this event is as tough as the first one. The departure from Newcastle is at noon, a far more respectable time of day to start, and we start in a far more relaxed frame of mind, having organised a pasta party the night before with a group of other riders. The atmosphere is buoyant as we set off, although the weather forecast for the day is not looking good; storms are predicted.

An hour into the ride, having got out of the city without incident, the cyclists have all stretched out. As usual I am near the back, watching rider after rider passing me and heading off into the distance. It's demoralising to see people disappearing ahead, calculating in my head that they will be in and out of the feed station before I am anywhere near it.

My mood is not improved as the growing dark clouds decide to let go of their load and heavy raindrops start to fall. As the miles slide by under my wheels, the rain gets heavier and heavier. The groups of bystanders who had been out on the streets as we left Newcastle are a distant memory. No one is out in this torrential weather to give us a cheer. The rain pours through the air vents in my crash helmet, soaking my head, and a steady stream of water runs down my nose and off my chin. I'm sure even ducks wouldn't go out in this heavy weather. I'm soaked to the skin. Thankfully I have packed two extra sets of dry cycle gear in my day bag, which will be waiting for me at each feed station.

With rain in my eyes, I am struggling up a hill, determined not to get off. With my feet tightly fixed to my pedals with cleats, there is a fine balance in knowing when to unclip. Sadly, I get it wrong. Pushing one extra turn of the pedals, I'm going at such a slow pace I am going to have to stop. But I cannot unclip my foot; rather than fall into the road in front of the passing traffic, I have no choice but to fall towards the pavement. Laying there on my left side, with both feet clipped into the pedals, in the pouring rain, I feel at my lowest. To add to my misery, as I pick myself up I realise I've taken a big chunk out of my left knee as I hit the kerb. There are no other riders around and no support vehicle; all I can do is ride on to the next feed station with blood pouring down my leg.

Patched up, I head back out into the storm. Whilst Lucie and I had signed up to take on this ride as a relay team, at the last moment we had done our maths and reckoned we could both do it solo. This meant after each 15-minute rest stop we had to get back in the saddle and take on the next 45- to 50-mile stretch. After three stints, it is clear that this weather is going to beat us. We were perhaps a little foolish to change our plan at the last minute, and we change back to doing it in relay. We are both getting worn down by the continuous rain. As we do a relay swap, I take the time to warm up and change into a dry set of cycle kit as I get transported to the next changeover. We're not the only ones struggling, as the bus has to pick up riders who are battling against the weather.

Despite the rain, I am pleased that my stoma bag routine is working. With the weather forecast, I was concerned that with my skin being so wet for so long, maybe the adhesive on my base plate would come unstuck. But, so far, all is well. My night stint falls at 3am. The rain has temporarily stopped, and by now a small group of us have buddied up. None of us wanted to ride through the night alone, so we formed a pact that we would ride together and stay together, even if one of us had a puncture. There's no support out there to help in these circumstances, so we are in it together.

Perhaps it's the heady mix of fatigue and adrenaline, but as we weave between giant puddles, and ride through the middle of the roads that have flooded over completely, our laughter breaks into song. We are riding through the remote countryside around the Peterborough area, so there's no one to hear us. The companionship of strangers makes the riding seem so much easier, and we pick up some waifs and strays along the way.

At the final feed station, Gethin is having to pull out due to injury and James has gone ahead. Lucie is exhausted and talking about pulling out. As rider after rider leave on their final stretch into north London, we chat about what we have achieved so far together and how our husbands and children will be there at the finish line waiting for us. We've just got to push hard this one last time. The rain has finally stopped, and we change into our final set of dry clothes. From Royston in Hertfordshire, our mood is lifted as the sun comes out. Heading south gives us a mental feeling of it being all downhill. Lucie and I are riding this last stage together, side by side. Riding through the north London traffic, we make our last final turns into the sports ground and see the finish line. We've made it together and cross the line hand in hand. Not only has my body survived another 24-hour event, it's endured some of the toughest weather we could ever imagine. Who says a stoma is going to hold me back? What more could I achieve?

Chapter Six

SITTING POOLSIDE, I hold my breath as Robert and Natasha have their swimming lessons in the deep end. Both began swimming from the age of five with the Ilfracombe Swimming Club; Craig and I felt it was crucial that our children must know how to swim, as we live by the sea. Personally, I've always been scared of the water from an incident when I was at primary school. I can flounder about in the shallow end, but my head is always so far above the water, it's like a submarine periscope. Getting my face wet or, even worse, putting my head underwater, either deliberately or accidentally, sends me into a panic attack, hyperventilating and getting out of the water in tears. I'm so proud of Robert and Natasha swimming like dolphins. More and more they ask Craig and me to go swimming with them, but I am always hesitant. So I have made up my mind that I need to learn to swim. Now that I am an active mum again, why should I let something in my head stop me from enjoying swimming with my children?

My first lessons at Ilfracombe Pool: I am so nervous. I've put on a new stoma bag to make sure it has well and truly stuck to my skin; I know they are designed for everyday wear and tear, and I wear it in the shower, but I've never had the confidence to get in a pool with it. I have treated myself to a pair of Aqua Sphere mask-like goggles, as they allow me good visibility. I feel really panicky with the little eye-socket style goggles. Lesson one is simply about building confidence in the water. The swim teacher tells our small group to bob down low enough for our mouths and noses to be underwater and to blow bubbles. How easy is this? Fantastic. Gradually we can put our heads down under the water, still practising our blowing bubbles out slowly. To begin with, I naturally hold my breath and feel the panic rising, but, doing this at my own pace, I find that the panic subsides as the air gently leaves my lungs. Watching the bubbles rise to the surface in front of my goggles, I am reassured that if I need to breathe, the surface is right there.

As the weekly lessons pass, we start to be led down towards the deep end. So far, I've been quite comfortable as we have stayed in the shallow end. We've been diving down to swim through hoops, which had initially been held just below the surface, but were then lowered down to the floor level at the shallow end. We have also been practising the front crawl. My brain cannot seem to remember everything at the same time. I can get the arm movement going, but forget to kick and totally mess up the breathing. We are trying to breathe on every third stroke, and it's a struggle. I do make progress, however, and I am happy that I can now swim from the wall to halfway down the length of the pool. Going to the deep end brings back my nerves. I sidle along holding the edge of the pool until we are a little deeper, and the teacher gets us to swim from this point back to the shallow end.

SIX

In two months, I have got my confidence and can swim a couple of lengths of the pool; my face is in the water and I am getting the breathing right now. When I started I couldn't swim at all, but gradually I have built up the stamina to swim two lengths, even if I do stop for a breather at the end of the lane each time. Taking a break over Christmas, I get that itch for a new challenge. Swimming has reignited my desire to set a goal. I know I can ride a bike, I know I can swim and running is easy for anyone. I know ... I'll have a look at triathlons. With that I find my local triathlon club, the North Devon Triathletes, and I sign up to be a member. If I want to be a triathlete, then I have to train with triathletes.

The club meet at Barnstaple swimming pool every Sunday at 9am. I don't know anyone, but one thing I have never lacked is the confidence to walk into a room and speak to complete strangers. Now I am walking up to a group of experienced triathletes, armed only with a swim cap and a pair of goggles. I am feeling very exposed in my swimming costume, but I feel confident that no one can see my stoma bag through it. During my swimming lessons, I found that the base plate, on to which my stoma bag clips, was getting really 'gummy'; it never came unstuck, but it definitely left a sticky mess after I got out of the pool.

When I left hospital after my surgery, I was given some stoma supplies, and I had continued with them ever since. However, part of learning to live with an ostomy is realising that there is so much choice out there. The stoma care nurses can only provide you with so much, but once you get online and visit some stoma care group events, you get to see and try products that you never realised were available.

The issue with water on the base plate (flange) of my stoma bag was my biggest problem, so I requested samples from all the different stoma supply companies to see which worked best. Not only did I come across a product that didn't absorb water like the hydrocolloid base I had been using, I also came across some silicone flange extenders from a company called Trio Ostomy Care, whose products are all based on silicone. These are like a fine skin that I can put on over the edge of my flange, and there is absolutely no way any water gets under there. These are a dream find for what I need.

At the tri club, I am warmly welcomed and I join the first lane, which is where the slightly weaker swimmers are grouped together. The club takes up four lanes at this time in the morning, and there's a large proportion of super-fit-looking men in the other three lanes. I'm feeling rather intimidated and a little excited at being in the water with these guys. The training is hard, so much tougher than I'm doing in my lessons. I have continued with my swimming lessons during the week, even though I have joined the tri club. I have progressed from the beginners' group up to the intermediate group. Being with the triathletes, I am totally out of my league, but putting into practice what I have learned in the week is paying dividends. Being with others who are new to this is reassuring, and we all have to up our swimming just to be here. From being just about able to swim two lengths, this feels like a marathon!

After a few weeks of regular attendance, the man teaching us from the poolside has decided to mix in some swim exercises in pairs. One swimmer holds the ankles of the other. Whilst the swimmer on the front uses their arms to do the front crawl, the person on the back does the kicking. I am teamed up with one of the men. I am nervous

SIX

at the thought of this – I cannot even get my breathing every third stroke exactly right yet. As we set off, I am put on the back. Holding the ankles of this chap, I am a weak kicker and I am sure I am holding him back. He's pulling away with his arms, but his legs are sinking because he cannot kick. As his legs sink, my arms are sinking with them, and with it my head is underwater more and more and I am being dragged along; I cannot breathe, I cannot get my head up for air. I panic. I let go of his legs just halfway down the pool and turn back to the end of the lane, apologising to him. I climb out in tears. I cannot do this. Who do I think I am, being able to swim with these guys? I leave them to finish off, embarrassed at sitting on the side of the pool crying. I may feel broken, but I won't be beaten, so join the rest of the lesson in the slow lane.

* * * * *

With the support of my new-found friends at the tri club, I am starting to get out and do more regular training. The Sunday swim is now routine for me, and on Saturdays I can either head out for a bike ride with some of the ladies in the group, or join in with the Barnstaple Park Run. These are free events organised locally, with 5km timed runs. The camaraderie of around 100 runners at all levels is great motivation. So much for me thinking that 'running is easy for anyone': it really isn't easy. It's my weakest discipline, as I just cannot keep running – I have to regularly switch to walking.

This particular Saturday morning, there is a large contingent of the tri club members taking part. There's a big national awareness of Park Run taking place, and we are expecting a lady called Chrissie Wellington to be attending ours; then she's going down to the beach with the tri club to do some sea swimming. As a total newcomer to triathlon, I confess this name means nothing to me, but clearly everyone is very excited about her coming. I'm told she is a four-time Ironman world champion.

She is such a down-to-earth lady when we all meet her. She shares with us a little about her dream of triathlon and what it's taken for her to consistently become a world champion. Her story strikes a chord with me. From being a runner with a day job, being hit by a car, and then coming back to take on triathlon on a third-hand Peugeot: this woman has fought for what she wants and has dedicated herself to her sport to achieve the highest ambitions. At that moment I am acutely aware of what I've been through to just get to this point in time – to be able to take part in a 5km Park Run, to be able to swim and to have completed two 24-hour cycle events. Here is a woman who is the epitome of who I want to be: a fighter with a cause. She leads out the 5km run, beating everyone of course, and I am humbled to be running the same course with her, even if it is just our local Park Run. My mind is set: I want to become a real triathlete, one that competes at all levels. I've always watched the tough endurance sports on television and seen grown men struggle to finish an Ironman course. That's the ultimate goal, but I am going to have to work my way up to that level. Nothing comes without hard work, and juggling home and work with training is always tough. Even if all I do is shorter distances, I know I can be a triathlete.

* * * * *

As it turns out, my first attempt at taking part in a triathlon is at our in-club tri held at Holsworthy in March 2015. It's not an official event, more of a pre-season warm-

SIX

up for everyone, and a large number of the club take part. Roughly a sprint distance event, it's a 500m pool swim, 21km bike and 6km run.

The week before the event, a small number of club members meet up to ride the route, so we've got an idea of where we are going. I am clearly the slowest of the group, and club member James Marshall, who has organised the triathlon, gives everyone clear instructions for the route and sticks with me, as I am just holding everyone else up. He tells me not to worry about everyone else and to just stick to a pace that I can work to in order to get round.

A week later, I am a bag of nerves. I know pretty much everyone here now, and yet I'm terrified of what I am about to do. I set up my bike along the railings outside the pool with my box of clothes, shoes, helmet and gels ready for the bike stage. Craig and the children have come along to watch me race, which is reassuring and a chance for them to meet my tri club friends. In the changing rooms, my legs are like jelly. I am reminded that this is just our in-club event and there's no pressure. As I am a slow swimmer, I am one of the first into the lanes. Have I remembered everything? Thankfully I am not the only nervous newcomer, and the girls either side of me wish me luck, as I do for them. As the horn goes, I push off from the wall and get into a rhythm. My breathing technique is pretty much every third stroke and I am pleased with this, but I am still left breathless and have to take a short moment's break at the end of every length. I see the ladies either side of me stretching ahead. I'm counting the lengths and relieved when I see the board in the water from the marshal, indicating that I am now about to swim my last two lengths. By now, new swimmers have joined the lanes either side of me and I know I am falling behind.

Out of the pool, I run out to my bike. I'm worried I am going to be cold out there in a wet trisuit, so I pull up my cycle shorts and endeavour to put on my long-sleeve cycle jersey. Lesson number one: legs and arms do not slide easily into clothing whilst wet! I battle with my clothes for an eternity as the club members simply hop on to their bikes and are off. I sit down to dry off my feet and fight with my socks, which are resisting being shoved on to damp toes. Eventually, suitably togged up, I am off on the bike. At least I know the route from last week, which I am grateful for. There are fewer and fewer people on the road in front of me and more and more coming past. In the saddle, I am happy that I have completed the swim and now there's only this and the run to go.

Back into the pool car park that is doubling up as our transition area, I peel off the cycle shorts and change into my running shoes. Just the run now. I've done this at Park Run: easy! Heading out, I'm getting high-fived and cheered on by fellow club mates who are on the return journey. There's no cheating with this out-and-back run; they've written a phrase on the back of the board at the turning point, and we have to say it when we finish. Along the road isn't too bad, but I'm doing my normal run/walk approach on the flat. I follow the arrows down a country lane, and this is predominantly a downhill run, which isn't too bad. In fact, I am getting too hot with my long-sleeve jersey on, and I've taken to running with it in my hand. As Ian Hindes, one of our fast runners, comes by me, he offers to take it back to the finish line for me. That's great – it's freed me up.

I see no one else: absolutely everyone has gone past me, turned and gone back the other way. I now know I am absolutely last and I am not even at the halfway point

SIX

yet. From behind me comes a voice; James Marshall runs alongside me, encouraging me. 'Not far now to the turn point,' he says. James is actually the guy who is running round to collect up the signs. Yep, I am that slow: even the clearer-upper has caught me! I'm getting cold now, as I am not moving quickly enough to keep warm. Not only does James instruct me on how to run a minute, walk a minute, he's also sacrificed his running top for me.

We get to the main road and turn off for the final loop of the park before the finish back at the pool.

'If you want to cut it short, Caroline, you can cut across the path in the park, rather than go all the way around,' he says.

'No way! I've come this far – I don't want to cut this at all.'

With that, I give him back his jersey, grateful for his help, and I run off on the final loop. Crossing the bridge from the park to the pool car park to the sound of cheering, I am over the moon – I've made it. I may be slow, but I have finished. Slow is an understatement: the final competitor before me had come over the finish line a whole 20 minutes earlier. I've got a lot of work to do, and today has proved to me that running is not my favourite or strongest discipline. But I have the determination to keep going. Having an ileostomy will not stop me.

* * * * *

This morning started on a real high. I recently bought *Swim Workouts for Triathletes*, and this morning I set about the first programme in the book. The warm-up alone took me half an hour before I even got to the main set. Whilst I only had an hour before work, I felt like a real professional with my fins, kickboard and pullbuoy sets. I may not have finished the programme today (as I am not quick enough to complete it within the hour), but I still managed 2.2km.

Recently I have buddied up with a fellow triathlete from the North Devon Tri Club to train together. Al is relatively new to the club and was looking for someone to train with at an equal level. Considering my level isn't great, I fit the bill. Over the last three weeks, we have chatted via Facebook about the events in 2016 and a training plan. There is nothing more motivating than to train with someone and then race together.

However, even though we have yet to hit the road together, he has just found out his job is taking him abroad from the end of January. I feel like the rug has been pulled from under me before we've even started. This morning I was on a high from training, and now I've lost my buddy. He won't be racing in the UK next year, so not only will we not be able to train together, we won't race together either.

I have suggested we do our 'virtual training' together over the internet. We're both competitive and it will be fun – but not the same. The sweetener is that there is a Half Ironman distance race near where he's moving to, and he's welcomed me and a load of our fellow tri club members over there next October to race.

A week later, and it's a damp and dreary morning, and I'm struggling to get up! So much for my plan to head over to the Barnstaple Park Run for 9am! It's funny how the weather affects your mood. I guess this is where having a proper training plan and structure in place kicks in and I do what I have to do regardless of the weather.

Up and about, I see a Facebook post from Al, who's out in Reims with a cold beer. I tell him how grotty the

SIX

weather is and that I'm dithering about going out for a run. 'Go run, Caroline,' he says. 'No slacking.' This is just the kind of kick up the backside I need, and I head out into the rain.

Thinking the old railway line was a 'nice flat run' was so wrong. Heading out, it has a deceptive incline, so no wonder my run feels slow and heavy. This fat belly of mine needs to improve. After slogging to the 2.5km mark with intermittent walks and runs, I find the return journey so much better – it's all downhill. In total I cover 5.7km in 39 minutes. That's not too bad after all, and the sun has come out. The only downside of this country lane run is that I've been bitten by a horsefly. I hate horseflies – I react really, really badly to them!

The bite on my hand has caused it to swell up. Packing it with ice helps to numb the irritation, but that's about all. I wonder if having a compromised immune system from ulcerative colitis means I now react badly to these?

* * * * *

As the summer months roll by, I find I am spending more and more time on the bike than on the other disciplines. Swimming I am coming to enjoy, and running is still my nemesis. It's easy for us to turn to the things we enjoy best and put off the things that we struggle with. When I was ill I would 'put off' the discussions about potentially having stoma surgery, and yet here I am doing things I never thought I could do and would never have taken up before I had that life-changing moment. If I had never pushed myself to have swimming lessons to enjoy time with my children, I would never have turned to triathlons, but when something major occurs in your life, it changes you. You can let that be a change for the worse, or you can embrace the change: recognise that things will never be the same, and make the most of what you do have.

I've signed myself up for yet another charity cycle event. This is not quite as intense as the 24-hour events I started out on, but is ridden over a number of days.

Ride for Precious Lives is a ride of 205 miles across three counties in three days, visiting each of the three children's hospices of Children's Hospice South West: Little Harbour near St Austell, Little Bridge House near Barnstaple, and Charlton Farm near Bristol. With a target of around 65 to 80 miles each day, the North Devon Tri Club enter a team of eight: Graham Salisbury, Sarah Logan, Mark Rhead, Donna Marriott, Tina Kiff-Jamieson, Shelley Hadley, Susan Standford and myself, plus two honorary members for the trip, Elizabeth Mason and my Newcastle to London team-mate Lucie Gallen.

On day one, the excitement of being out together as a team goes to our heads. The iconic NDT cycle jerseys are prevalent on the road, and there's a special camaraderie from cycling together with a common goal. We are raising money for a worthy cause, doing something we are all passionate about. A couple of the team push out ahead at a faster pace, whilst the rest of us do our best to keep a good speed. There are moments where we become separated as a few take wrong turns, so some extra miles of backtracking are required to regroup.

The event has a euphoric feel to it, riding through some of the most stunning scenery. We ride across moors dotted with wild ponies, through hills and flat terrain. We stop on the top of Exmoor to 'twerk' to Heart FM, which is playing 'We Are the Champions' from its support car for us. Along the way our little group collects some extras

SIX

who are riding in ones and twos and struggling along on their own. Our happy band grows, and, with it, the joy of riding is enhanced.

One by one we all tackle the climb up through Cheddar Gorge, waiting at the top to cheer every rider through. By the final day, we are riding like a machine. The terrain is predominantly flat and we get a chain going, where the rider at the front sets the pace for a few minutes, creating a wind-free tunnel for the chain of riders behind them. They peel off and drop to the back of the chain, where the new leader takes the brunt of the wind resistance. Circulating like this, the chain picks up speed, and we make great time and feel like a professional peloton. What freedom. Even the puncture at the gates of the driveway to our final destination doesn't dampen our spirits. We started as a team and we will finish as a team. We are the last team home, but we make sure to turn it into a Tour de France-style roll-in.

* * * * *

The support I receive from the North Devon Tri Club is second to none. Having finished the in-club tri earlier in the year, I feel like I have 'earned my stripes' and can call myself a triathlete. Just a few months ago, I knew none of these fantastic people and was just another newcomer. But we all have different abilities, and whilst only one or two of the girls now know about my ileostomy, one thing we all have in common is the desire to improve and to compete, and I truly appreciate the encouragement the other triathletes give me to try my best. I've already overcome my fear of water in a pool, but the thought of swimming in open water is a whole different realm of fear for me. I know that at some stage I am going to have to try this too, but if I can just do pool swims, then I am happy with that.

I appreciate that I'm no professional when it comes to triathlons, and my swimming is not particularly fast – I like to think that I am built for endurance, not speed (so I keep telling everyone). When I started my first forays into triathlons, I came across a man who had done Ironman events in his younger years and obviously believed he was well placed to coach others.

I admit he can help me to focus on technique, and, in the early days of talking to him, this was great. I was part of a small group who he shouted instructions out to from the poolside. However, now he is more often in the water and swims with the fast boys and doesn't 'coach' so much. Last week, using my new swim workout book, I would say I had my best training session in ages. This swim session with the 'boys', though, was the complete opposite. I decided to join his Tuesday group at 7am and found myself put in a lane with three 12-year-old lads, whilst the other older swimmers had the other lane. I don't have a problem being in a 'slower' lane and swimming with the supposedly slower youngsters, but these three boys had no pool etiquette. As they passed me in their dash to beat one another, they would swim over my arms, kick me as they cut back in front of me, and cut me up at the end of the lane, just as I was about to turn. Who's teaching them the manners that come with swimming with others in a lane? I am the only woman in this swimming session, and I am feeling particularly pushed aside.

The 'coach' clearly wasn't educating these lads or even correcting what they were doing. In the end I made my excuses of having to get to work, and got out of the pool early after only having swum 950m. That's not even half

SIX

what I'd done the previous week on my own. I'm definitely not one to think I know it all and I am definitely no professional swimmer, but I have learned to respect the abilities of others in the pool.

My time with this 'coach' is over – he seemed to wash his hands of me when I couldn't commit to swimming at 6.30am three times a week. He would take us all down to the local beach to practise in open water, and, even knowing that I was only just overcoming a fear of water, he just kept shouting for me to put my face in the water. I just couldn't do it. In the pool, the water is clear and I can see around me, but in the sea it is dark and murky with no visibility, and the fear just washes over me again.

I am never going to be a professional triathlete, and it's unlikely that I will ever make it to any kind of podium position. I'm a middle-aged mum with a husband, two kids and a business to run – triathlon is a hobby that I enjoy, so it's time to put the overbearing style of coaching behind me and get on with focussing on my own training that fits with my lifestyle.

Chapter Seven

MY HEART is pounding so hard – I haven't felt like this since going into surgery to have my large intestine and colon removed. The feeling I have today is *exactly* like I felt as I was laid on the surgeon's table with a team of nurses around me.

I was truly scared beyond belief about being knocked out and having such major surgery. I recall being tearful then, feeling alone, knowing that I had to go through this. The nurse assured me that my anaesthetist was looking after me. She held my hand until who knows when. ... I just passed out.

Today I am sat at my computer screen waiting for the Ironman registration to open. I have found that popular events sell out almost immediately, and if I don't grab the opportunity, even if I am committing to a cost without having a sponsor to cover it, the window of opportunity might be closed and then I'd regret hesitating.

As the minutes tick by, the words on the screen change from 'Opening Soon' to 'Open'. I click on the 'register' button and start to fill out my details – that's when my heart starts thumping.

SEVEN

'Am I doing the right thing?' 'Am I really just being stupid and pretending I could ever be an Ironman?' 'Can I really commit to this entrance fee when I have scraped every penny I could spare together?'

I get to the final page, where I fill in my bank card details. At the bottom is the very final 'SUBMIT' button. I hesitate. I think of what I have achieved in the last 18 months since taking up triathlons; I think of all my fellow ostomates who have such belief in me. I cannot give myself an excuse to not do something I have dreamed of for so long. I hit the button!

What have I done? Registration is confirmed. I am now entered into Ironman Bolton 2016. Tears spring to my eyes – just like they did on the surgeon's table six years ago.

* * * * *

Having others around you who watch you grow, encourage you and support you is crucial in any personal development. After my surgery, it took a while before I started to reach out and speak to people about my stoma. In those first days and weeks, my biggest concern was about going out in public. What if I needed to change my bag in a public toilet? It was all such a rigmarole. It was Robert and Natasha who actually made it easier for me to come to terms with this. I'd have to use a large disabled cubicle just to get me and both children in, but the kids were fascinated by my stoma and even called it 'strawberry', because, to them, that's what it looked like.

Their matter-of-fact acceptance made me question what I was worrying about. If I didn't eat for a while, my stomach would get gassy and my stoma would emit the gas into the bag. The children thought this was hilarious – strawberry farts in a bag.

I find a closed Facebook group called Ostomy Lifestyle Athletes (OLA). Every person in this group has an ostomy of one description or another, and yet they are getting out and enjoying their lives with sport. These are definitely my kind of people. They become my 'go to' place for questions, and it is inspiring to hear they are ultra-runners, obstacle course competitors, bodybuilders, pole dancers, rugby players, elite cyclists and even American wrestlers. Some people in the group enjoy the less extreme sports like swimming, walking, jogging, kayaking and Zumba classes. Never have I met such a positive, uplifting group of global individuals.

They are the first place I go after hitting the 'register' button for Ironman. They are delighted for me and tell me they know I can do this. One of the guys, Marc Mahoney, lives in the Bolton area and is even making sure he is a marshal on the event to cheer me round, and has offered to take me out to ride the bike course in advance. What a fantastic support team I have, and the majority of them I have never even met face-to-face. There is a special bond between us.

Next I tell Al, my training buddy. He doesn't yet know my surgical history, but tells me I have guts for entering. How funny that people say I've got guts, when in reality I don't have any at all. How ironic!

By taking on a challenge like this, I know I can inspire others, and I want to be a role model to my children – showing them that anything is possible if you put your mind to it and dedicate the time and effort required for success. But I am also doing this for myself. This sport has shown me what I am capable of, and I wish I'd found it when I was much younger. I am bloody-minded and stubborn, so I am told, and I realise that I need to be in order to compete in triathlons. I will never expect to be on a podium, but I can see myself being stronger and improving. I am going to be 50 next month, yet I feel like I am in my 30s.

* * * * *

Isn't it strange how the perception others have of you can be so different to how you perceive yourself? This morning, Al and I swam together for the first time. To date, Al has made me feel very important; he has put me on a pedestal – although I have told him it should be more like a footstool! He wanted to find a training partner of a somewhat similar pace and approached me. I am flattered, and his remarks do make me look back at how I have come on with my training over the last 18 months. From feeling like the newbie who needs a coach, I now feel like the coach. Al sees me as his motivator, and I hope that by sharing our training I don't let him down.

Recently when we were chatting, he said he had heard all about me from Kimberley 'Kimbo' Pickett – one of the ladies in the tri club – and he was very impressed. He had never told me what she had said, and I assumed she had mentioned my ileostomy. Now, this lady in the tri club is someone who I really admire – a relative newcomer too, she is very dedicated to her training, and I wish I could be like her.

Today, however, Al told me he hadn't known about my stoma; what Kimbo had told him was 'Caroline's really impressive; she's a machine.' I am totally overwhelmed and chuffed to bits at her perception of me. Clearly what I do in my eyes seems somewhat lacking, but to those around me it is amazing and inspirational. So now I want to make sure that in whatever I do, I inspire others. I am still a newbie at this, yet I have obviously made an impression on my peers. I look forward to the next training session with Al. To me, we are equals.

* * * * *

After a week's holiday – camping, of all things – I am feeling sluggish and 'can't be bothered'. All I have done is eat rubbish food – burgers, fish and chips, pizzas – and I'm really feeling the impact on my body. I am not fanatical about food and have a generally healthy diet, but this week I have 'blobbed out' and now feel bloated and lethargic.

Camping is something I've not done for many years. In my youth I remember it was full of mud and 'roughing it', but now my children want to experience living in the great outdoors and there is that desire in me to get out there with them. When I was ill, there was no way on earth I would have gone out and slept in a tent, and there is a nervousness about camping now with my ileostomy. What if I have a bag leak in my sleeping bag? What if I cannot find a toilet with a sink handy? This is the first holiday since that disastrous trip to Butlins when I spent the whole week in the chalet.

I needn't have worried so much. With my ileostomy, I just have a few extra things to consider. I was a bit dubious about the thought of having to deal with my stoma in the confined space of a tent, but in reality the gnats that thought I was a walking feast were a far bigger problem. All it takes is a little bit more forward planning. The first campsite had a 'pitch where you like' approach, which was ideal as it meant we could pitch up close to the shower block. Now, my body has a night-time routine all of its

SEVEN

own; I knew that I would wake up some time around 4am and need to deflate the 'hot air balloon' that is my stoma bag (yes, they fill with gas as well as output!). So planning to be close to the toilet block was ideal. I had my bag of stoma products, my jacket, a torch and wellies sat in the corner of the tent ready for my night-time trip. It was just like getting up in the night at home, except I don't usually choose to wear wellies to go to the bathroom.

Blobbing out back at home and with just a couple of weeks to the Ilfracombe Triathlon, I have decided to get up early today and cycle the tri route. I know it's hilly, and, having not done any cycling for the last three weeks, I know this could be a 'toughie'. The plan was: wake at 7am, grab breakfast and be out by 8am for the ride, which should take about 90 minutes to cover 16 hilly kilometres. In reality it turns out to be: alarm goes off at 7am, keep hitting the snooze button until 7.30am, drag myself out of bed, get breakfast, dig out my bike clothes and get ready to go. But then I remember I have left the bike at the office, 12 miles away! What a dope! Rather than stomping around in frustration, I decide to go for a run instead.

I am really not that keen – my running can be a slog, but I might as well go, otherwise all I ever do is make excuses for not going, then regret it later on when I know that had I pushed myself, my running would be so much better. Practice makes perfect – at least, in my case, practice makes it more achievable even if it will never be perfect.

A short walk from the house turns to a gentle jog, and before I know it I am into a gentle stride all the way down to the harbour and I'm not even breathless. I decide I will do the Ilfracombe Triathlon run route this morning. Having competed last year, I know that the run route is a hard cliff-face climb. I haven't been up here since the event last year, so know it's going to be hard today, but I could do with the practice. However, having competed in various triathlons in the last 12 months, my fitness is much better and I manage the route. I still have to walk up the steep cliff paths, but 'so what?' – I still make it. In total, I run 4.5 miles. I'm pleased with that!

I am now getting serious about competing in the full Ironman event – 2.4-mile swim, 112-mile bike and a marathon! Rather than just doing some sporadic sport training, I am actually setting a proper training programme to achieve my dream. I am planning my events so I can build my body to achieve the ultimate goal. I have booked Snowdonia Slateman Savage on 21 and 22 May 2016. This comprises racing a sprint triathlon on the Saturday – 500m open-water swim, 16km bike up Pen-y-Pass at Llanberis, and a 5km run up through woodland. The following day I will race the Olympic distance course (double the sprint lengths), but this time the run goes up through the slate quarries – that's why they call this 'Savage'. Running the cliff-faces and hills around Ilfracombe is therefore an ideal training ground for Slateman.

Then on 12 June, I am racing in the Ironman 70.3 (Half Ironman) in Staffordshire. This is notoriously hard (what triathlon isn't hard?), with a technical bike course and a hilly run route. The full Ironman in July is double the distances again. I cannot believe I'm even at the level of doing a local triathlon, yet here I am really pushing my personal boundaries.

* * * * *

This morning I had my local sprint triathlon. Last year I was terrified – I had never done a sea swim tri before and was really nervous. This year, however, I am feeling calm and relaxed. The sea is flat, and it's sunny. Having a chance to get into the water in the harbour and acclimatise helps, but I didn't have enough time to get my face down in the water, and that rush of sea water going down my wetsuit is so cold!

Despite this, I am still feeling more confident this year, and, rather than walk in at the back, I actually run into the sea. However, I am very conscious of others around me, in particular behind me, as I don't want anyone swimming over me. The water in the harbour is calm, but I'm not! Despite all the beautiful swimming I can do in the pool, out here I just cannot get my face in the water. My breathing is all over the place, but it's reassuring having someone on a paddleboard alongside me.

Even though I'm slow, I am still with the pack, albeit I am at the back. Once out of the harbour, the sea is more turbulent. On an incoming tide, the waves want to push me towards the rocks and I feel I'm going nowhere. I try to breathe on every second stroke, which means I keep seeing the rocks! This is tough! I focus on technique; I must stop flailing around and must relax. I feel my arms pull down through the water – catch, pull, back; I feel my thumbs touch my thigh – the focus helps me relax. I must relax and trust my training.

Out of the water and up to Transition One, my wetsuit slides off easily and I am on my bike before the lady next to me. A short, sharp climb and I am on to the bike route; I live here in Ilfracombe and know what's coming – it's a 5km climb: a long, long, long drag, but I get my rhythm and am comfortable. I don't care I'm near the back. I can hear my brake rubbing very slightly and stop to adjust it. There's still no sign of the last competitor!

Up on the flat for a while, then down a long technical descent; despite the sunshine, the wind-chill factor against my wet trisuit makes me feel cold. Some tough climbs take me back to transition. Whilst I am now putting on my shoes for the 6km run, the fast competitors have already finished! Ah well, I'm used to this.

The run is very steep, but to start with I have to get over the pain of 'jelly legs' from getting off the bike. What keeps me going is all the cheers, claps and words of encouragement from passers-by – this really does keep you going.

I finish in 2 hours, 53 minutes, 55 seconds.

* * * * *

A week later and my day is full of excitement for a couple of reasons. First, because I cycled from Bideford to Land's End and back (200 miles) for the local chemotherapy unit last September, I have been invited to attend the Royal Opening of the unit. Myself and my fellow cycling fundraisers are going to attend on our bikes, wearing the cycle jerseys we had specially designed for the occasion. We had hoped to raise £3,000 from our efforts, but the team actually hit £5,000.

This ride was first suggested by my friend Ed Johns, as his sister Jane (who is also a good friend) had been treated for cancer but had had to travel backwards and forwards to Exeter. So, when the North Devon District Hospital in Barnstaple was having a chemotherapy unit built, it was a very worthy cause that we wanted to be part of.

Six of us – Ed, Darrel Gill, Jayne Jarrett, Peter Quincey, Olly Keates and myself – planned our own event to cycle from Bideford in North Devon down to Land's End and back over a weekend, covering a total of 200 miles. It was a team effort to plan and organise, and we enlisted the help of friends to be our support team: Simon Grice, Simon Trow, Stephen Pitts and Diane Chaplin. We had a minibus, a mechanics van, a physiotherapist and a motorcycle outrider, all of whom were essential team members.

However, for me, disaster struck just five days before the event. Having dropped my bike in for a service, I'd opted to then run in to the office. Starting out at a gentle jog through the industrial estate, I was less than quarter of a mile from my start point when I stumbled and fell. Running along the pavement, approaching the entranceway to a builders' yard, I somehow lost my footing on the kerb, or maybe I just hadn't picked my feet up properly as I dropped down on to the road – but my legs went from under me in an instant, and my body slammed down on to the gravelly tarmac driveway. I'd twisted to my right as I fell, putting my hands out to save myself, but my right knee had taken the brunt of the fall.

I lay in the gutter stunned, unable to move. Shock froze me to the spot, and I couldn't move my right leg as early-morning commuters drove around me. Gradually putting my hands behind me to push myself up into a sitting position, I found myself surrounded by a couple of men from the builders' yard and a suited gentleman who had pulled over in his car to check I was all right. Stiffening up, my right knee was badly gashed open and blood was pouring down my leg. In an instant, the suited man whipped out a tissue to stem the bleeding; for someone dressed up for the office, the tissue was a kids' design, which made me smile – never judge people by their outward appearances!

The men from the builders' yard returned with a first aid kit and between them managed to bandage up my knee. As the suited man slowly helped me to my feet, it was clear I couldn't put any weight on my right leg, and he was a true saint when he offered to drive me to the hospital across town. His car was pristine and posh, and I sat very carefully in the front seat trying not to drip blood all over his carpet. Once I was dropped at A&E, I called Craig to let him know what had happened.

In the cubicle, a nurse cleaned up my wounds. The cut in my knee was deep and still bleeding. There was no other option but to stitch it up. Wearing my running gear, I explained to her what I was doing and even more so, my concern that in a week's time I was meant to be cycling from Bideford to Land's End and back. She looked at me with sympathetic eyes. Asked if there was a chance the stitches would be out by the end of the week, she hesitantly told me that the stitches really needed to stay in for ten days. Understanding my concern and the reason for my cycle event, she advised that I should see how the healing went over the week and get checked out a couple of days before the event. Only if the nurse thought it was OK would I be able to ride, but I shouldn't pin my hopes on that.

Desolate, I told the rest of the team what had happened.

Never had I been so good to follow the rules about rest and healing, so desperate was I to still be able to ride at the weekend. Two days before our big departure, I had my appointment with the nurse to review my knee.

'Sadly, Caroline, the stitches aren't really ready to come out. If you were to cycle all that way there's a very good chance that the wound would open up again.'

My face dropped – with my stubbornness and determination I had really thought I'd be able to get the

OK to ride. I knew it had only been a few days since the accident, but I was hoping for a miracle.

'If you're going to cycle 200 miles, I would suggest you keep the stitches in.'

With a glint in her eye, this nurse had just given me the almost-all-clear to ride! I could have hugged her! I'd have to keep the stitches in and keep the wound protected, but I could ride!

On the Friday morning, we set off from the quayside in Bideford to the waves and cheers of family and friends who have come out to see us go. The weather has been great, so we don't have to worry about getting soaked. Our target today is to ride to Newquay in Cornwall, where our first overnight stop will be. Relying on Jayne's navigation, we avoid as many of the main roads as possible for the sake of safety. Six cyclists in convoy with outriders can create a bottleneck on the narrower Devon roads. The scenery is fantastic and the camaraderie even better. We ride through Camelford and Wadebridge, stopping for regular food and drink top-ups, and roll into Newquay as the light is dropping after nearly 70 miles in the saddle.

Day two is tougher as the terrain gets even more hilly. Through Camborne and Hayle, we are getting closer and closer to our goal at the bottom of Cornwall. We cut across the county to Marazion for a lunch stop and some physiotherapy treatments, looking over the water at the iconic St Michael's Mount. We are all feeling the pain for miles in our legs and on our bums, but this location lifts our spirits. It's a good job it does, as the toughest is yet to come. Riding through Penzance, we head for Newlyn. Now, it's one thing looking at the profile of a route on a computer screen, but when you see what looks like a straight-up hill, that is something else! The hill is long and steep, and we've all agreed that everyone should take it at their own pace and wait at the top. With gritted teeth, we start the slog. Pete, Olly, Jayne and Ed start pulling away up the hill, whilst Darrel and I grind it out at a slower pace.

The legs are getting slower, the wheels are getting slower; if I don't get off now, then I am going to fall off, just like on Newcastle to London. I admit defeat. This is beyond me. As Simon picks up Darrel and me in the van and puts our bikes in the back, even the van is struggling to get up the hill. Only Peter makes it all the way to the top without stopping.

Psychologically, it feels like it's all downhill now. My knee is starting to hurt, but the adrenaline kicks in as we see Land's End ahead of us. It's full of tourists, and the six of us ride in together to the cheers of our support team. Dismounting under the iconic signage, my leg gives out. No more riding for me today, but I've made it this far.

Whilst the rest of the team ride back to St Ives, we reconvene and recover at Newquay for the final day tomorrow. Diane is kept busy with various niggles and injuries, and it's been fantastic having her 'mothering' us all with instructions on stretching and nutrition throughout the event. On the final day, we opt to use the wider main roads. We have the van and the motorcycle as our outriders so traffic can easily go around us. Having long, smooth tarmac roads, and legs that are on fire from over 140 miles, we absolutely fly! We reach our lunch stop at 11am – two hours ahead of ourselves. So we can afford a bit more rest. But still we keep gaining time. As we cross back into Devon, we know we are going to reach the finish early, so rushed phone calls are made to friends and family to be at Hartland Point earlier.

SEVEN

We group up outside Hartland for a bit of quiet personal time together as a group (and to repair the only puncture we've had) – we've bonded, and this is a special moment. All that's left is to ride down the hill to Hartland Point. Horns are blowing, and everyone is there to greet us. This is the most wonderful experience. I've competed in triathlons and taken part in cycling events, but this one is personal and means so much.

* * * * *

The second bit of excitement this morning is that I have heard that I am a semi-finalist in the Venus Businesswomen's Awards, in the Lifetime Achievement and Inspirational Woman of the Year categories. I am blown away by this, but my friends make me laugh, asking why I am so surprised. I do what I do because I can – before surgery, I had no choice, no life, no hope. I love the challenge, and the fact that I can raise money for charity doing it is just more motivation for pushing myself.

Taking up triathlons is definitely an expensive hobby. My old Peugeot Audax is a road bike designed for touring or long rides – it's no race bike. It's aluminium and therefore heavier than proper TT (time trial) bikes. I can build power in my legs, but with a lighter carbon fibre bike I could go quicker. Dream on, Caroline!

Well, dreaming was all I thought I could do – I cannot afford £2,000+ for a bike, plus new bike shoes and running shoes and all that paraphernalia. But at the Ilfracombe Triathlon, my friend Michelle Willcocks, who is also a triathlete with an ostomy, mentioned how she has had her travel expenses covered. Could I do that?

Well, reality is hitting me. I have made contact with Vanilla Blush, a company who make the most beautiful underwear and supportwear for ostomates, and they've come back to say potentially they and Trio Ostomy Care could sponsor me for a four-figure sum, which will cover all the items I need for upping my triathlon endeavours. This is serious stuff; I am so excited! A company is genuinely interested in my Ironman journey. I feel like a pro – just one phone call has turned around my thinking about this. This isn't a pipe dream any more – it's really happening. People believe in my challenge, my purpose; it's *really* happening! I just have to wait a few days to hear if this is going ahead. My poor brain has had so much excitement in one day. And to think, I was up at 5am to swim 2.2km before work; I'm shattered.

* * * * *

Blimey, I'm going to have to get used to these early starts. The clock was set for 4.45am. Today's plan is to meet Al at 6am so we can do a bike ride early before Park Run. As I get out of bed, I can hear the rain. Great, just great! But I know my training partner is going to be waiting for me, so I have to go. I am sure that if he wasn't going to be there, I'd just curl up back under my duvet for a few more hours.

At 6am, I park up at the agreed spot next to Al's van, and it seems to take forever to get myself ready. Lifting the bike out of the car, I obviously catch the quick release lever, and the front wheel drops off! Trying to get it back on in the semi-darkness is not easy.

As we prepare to leave, the rain begins again – not too much, but we put our wet gear on just in case. Ten minutes later, we are glad we did, as we are now soaked to the skin as the rain gets heavier and heavier. As we ride out on the eerily silent roads towards Bideford, we both admit that had it not been for the other, we wouldn't have headed out

SEVEN

into the rain. We keep pedalling hard as we cycle into the most horrendous headwind. We're out now, so we might as well just dig deep.

As we're turning away from the coast, the wind drops and we tackle the hills. Just when it seemed easier with the wind and rain, we get these hills! This is Al's choice of route and is clearly payback for the hard swim sessions I keep picking for us to do. He powers on up the hills ahead of me, but I know he will be waiting when I eventually get to the top.

The rain stops as we roll downhill to our start point. We drop the bikes off in our vehicles, peel off the top layer of our wet clothes and head to the start line of Park Run. Yes, this is our brick session day – 19.5 miles on the bike and 5km run. At least my run time for 5k, at 34 minutes, is only a few seconds off my usual pace, so clearly the soggy bike ride hasn't had any detrimental effect.

I head home feeling pleased with the efforts of the morning and am there by 10.30am, leaving the rest of the weekend clear to spend with my family. Fitting training in around family time is like an extra discipline. It takes organising to make sure my husband and children don't feel sidelined by my training, so I have always aimed to have Sundays as family day, except when I am racing, and I endeavour to get my Saturday training out of the way as quickly as I can.

Chapter Eight

EARLIER IN the year, with some encouragement from my North Devon Tri Club mates, I signed up to take part in the inaugural Tri the Beast triathlon, which is being held at Lynmouth. It's only a short distance away, so it seemed logical to participate in something right on my doorstep. But I also know it will be hard, as Lynmouth is at the bottom of a valley. To be honest, I know this is going to be a painful experience for me, as it is a sea swim and the course is so hilly. (You can tell by now that I am not keen on hills.) Heading down to the coast for the practice swim, a week before the event, I drive down a 25 per cent descent. Oh, joy – this is going to be a tough event.

Full of my 'gung-ho, I can do anything' attitude, I have rocked up a week before the event to participate in the swim practice that the organisers have laid on. Standing on the cobbled beach at the bottom of an enormous cliff-face, all I can see is a great expanse of sea. All my swimming has pretty much been in a pool, with just a very occasional dip in a sheltered cove near home. But, looking at where the buoys have been placed out at sea, I am immediately very scared.

EIGHT

Wetsuited up, I head to the water's edge with 24 others. This hour is to get us accustomed to the swim route in the sea. Getting into a rather turbulent sea, I sit down and let the cold seawater seep inside my wetsuit to acclimatise and rinse out my goggles. So far, so good.

We look to the first buoy far out to the right; from there we will swim parallel with the coastline to the second buoy, which is even further out to sea. Finally, we will have to turn and swim back inland. All my old fears kick back in as I find myself in tears. I am really struggling with sea swimming. I am frozen to the spot with fear; I cannot get down into the water and relax. I seriously cannot do this! My training is going well in the pool, but out here I go into panic mode.

Whilst 20 swimmers head off to go around the route, out to buoys that look miniscule they are so far out into the sea, I wade back to the shore to find I am not alone: three other ladies are in the same nervous state. It is only with the support of one of the organisers that we are all able to swim out to the nearest marker buoy (the last one on the course) and back again. Trying to overcome the panic and hyperventilation is so hard when there is nothing but sea in all directions and I cannot touch the floor. The organiser swims beside me, talking and reminding me to breathe. Bubble. Bubble. Breathe. Bubble. Bubble. Breathe. I am getting there; I just have to relax.

To swim to this marker buoy and back is a major achievement; I am disappointed that I didn't swim the course, but in that panicky state I would never have felt like I could get my breath. I am just going to have to trust my training and the advice of this swim coach. I know I can do this if I can just relax in the water – but I have my doubts for next weekend, when I have to swim this whole route.

It's nearly the end of the triathlon season, and I've only got this one more race to do. Sod's law says it's probably going to be the toughest Olympic distance I am ever likely to do. So, it's time to have some fun.

Having started to work at my core disciplines, I've signed up for a 5km run at Arlington Court on 24 October with some of my tri club buddies. It's advertised as a spooky run (race). We are all going to dress up – in fact, I'm probably going to face-paint us all as zombies. I've gone online to sign up for what I reckon will be a fun event, but there is actually a disclaimer on the sign-up page that is making me nervous. It warns anyone with a heart condition not to take part ... surely anyone with a heart condition is not likely to be running 5km! Anyhow, the reason for this warning is that in the dark woods, there will be zombies, axemen and the like, that will endeavour to scare us and make us think they are going to kill us! Oh, blimey – this now sounds really scary; the organisers have already sown that seed of doubt in my head.

I'm not a fast runner – my personal best is only 34 minutes 4 seconds for 5km – yet I have a feeling that I am likely to run through these woods so damned fast, I will smash my personal best. My team-mates had better not desert me out there. I wonder if I could tie myself to someone so they don't leave me behind?

I know it's just a bit of fun and I'm not really going to be killed, but the thought of zombies and people with axes coming at me out of the dark is really rather terrifying. Maybe I should have been looking for a bubble run instead.

* * * * *

It's been an emotional couple of days when I look back. I wonder whether this comes from the lack of training?

EIGHT

For two days prior to Sunday's Tri the Beast, I have been tapering – which essentially means resting up. I never thought I would actually miss training; after all, I am fundamentally lazy and in the past have found it hard to motivate myself to go out and train, so any excuse not to go out was great. But now I find I am itching to go out. Usually on a Friday I would swim around 3km before work. On Friday this week, I had to visit Bike It in Barnstaple to pick up some gels and energy bars for Sunday's race. Whilst I was there, the salesman, Lance, brought out a carbon fibre bike for me to see – a beautiful Giant Envie Advanced. In the past I would look at these bikes and admire them, but now I find myself talking seriously about the advantages of the bike and buying it! If I can only get a sponsorship deal signed up, this is the bike I am going to buy. Lance is a keen cyclist and gives me so much advice – it's wonderful to talk to him as an equal.

The bike is truly beautiful, and I can feel myself choking up! Why am I feeling so emotional towards a bike? It's not natural! This bike epitomises how far I have come in the last few years since my illness. It's professional, for serious competitors. Even considering riding this bike makes me feel like someone who's been training all their life. But when would I be in a position to ride it? A middle-aged woman about to turn 50, with no guts and a 'bag for life'.

* * * * *

Sunday is race day. Again, I find I am viewing these events differently these days. Just calling it 'race day' ... I know I am never going to be first at any of these events, but rather than just taking part, like in a sportive, I am very aware that this is a 'race'. If I am ever going to get anywhere close to a podium (in my age group), I am going to have to train very hard.

It's pitch black as I turn up at 6am; there's a beautiful silence across the picturesque town of Lynmouth and there's moonlight still low on the sea. A few street lights add a soft glow to the place, and as the early competitors arrive there is a gentle hum of voices, as if everyone is whispering whilst it's still dark. As the sun rises, so does the number of competitors. This is an inaugural event, so only 97 people have registered to give it a 'tri'. I am doing it because it's local and I know the area, but other competitors have driven down from all over the UK to compete.

The time for the race briefing on the beach seems to come around much quicker than expected. With a small number of us, it seems more relaxed. My fear of the swim, however, is palpable and I try my best to focus on the bike and run stages.

Wetsuit on and K-Y Jelly rubbed on both the inside and outside of my wetsuit arms and legs (for speedy stripping), I wander down to the stony shoreline. The beach at Lynmouth Bay is quite shallow, and we have to wait until the tide is in. It's going to be a floating start, whereby we all have to tread water before the horn goes off. Getting into the water, loads of us are stumbling over boulders under the shallow water whilst the gentle waves still knock us over. The hilarity of ourselves stumbling and bumping along on our bottoms sweeps aside the fear, and the laughter takes the pressure off.

I let some water into my wetsuit to acclimatise. It's not too cold, and I make my way over to the start buoy. I cannot believe it – we can actually all still stand up a good distance from the shore! Having those few minutes to

EIGHT

get out to the start buoy gives me time to calm down and check that my goggles aren't leaking. Last week I panicked in here, but today I'm determined to get round. Looking out along the coast to the first marker buoy, I tell myself that's the finish line – there's no better way to play with your head than to lie to yourself. Being at the back, I have a kayak paddling alongside me. This is reassuring and he's very encouraging.

Two hundred metres in and I can see a red swim cap ahead of me. I am usually accustomed to seeing them all disappear into the distance, but seeing someone else in front of me makes me realise I can't be doing too badly.

The red cap ahead has gone around the first buoy as I reach the turn point; my rhythm is starting to kick in; my breathing has calmed down and my face is now three-quarters into the water – definitely not all the way under like it would be in a pool, but I'm getting there.

As I reach the second marker buoy at the furthest point out at sea, I am feeling like I am in my stride. Round the buoy, and now I can see two red swim caps in front of me. We're heading inland for the flags on the beach, and the tide is helping to push us in. As we reach the shallows, I pass both the red caps! I cannot believe this: I've actually caught two people up on the swim discipline. I'm feeling elated to be out, and doing so much better than I thought I would.

Transition is slow, because I need to get as much gravel from the beach off my feet as I can, as there is now a gruelling bike ride and run.

The bike course is 29 miles of hills – and I mean big, steep hills. Wearing a wet trisuit when the sun hasn't yet shone through, it's rather chilly; maybe I should have put a cycle jersey on over the top? The bike stage begins with a three-mile climb up alongside Watersmeet. A long, steady grind I can do, but the steep switchbacks at the top are just too much for me and I have to walk for a bit. Riders doing the middle distance pass me – they had to swim two laps. At least I don't 'feel' like I am last, even if they are passing me.

The ride is, as I expected, gruesome: really evil hills. I get off at another steep switchback between Challacombe and Simonsbath, as I missed dropping down the gears so it's either unclip or fall off! At the top, we cross into Somerset, heading over the cattle grids and over the moors. I know now that I'm at the highest point and there's a seven-mile descent to transition. The roads across the moors are beautiful – long and sweeping, with only the sky above. Fingers crossed none of the sheep up here plan on crossing in front of me. I find when I am in remote beautiful locations like this that I talk to myself; I congratulate myself on getting up here. I'm sure if there was anyone else around, they would think I am mad!

The road starts to wind downward – sharply. In fact, the descent is as tough as the climbs for other reasons. I cannot just let the bike go; the bends are sharp and technical, so I am down on my drop bars with my hands on the brake levers. I am so glad I had new brakes put on the bike this week. My shoulders are burning from the position, but it's better than my legs screaming at me.

I'm on the final descent down Watersmeet, and I glance at my watch – it's only just gone 11am; this whole race started at 8am. That means (for me) I am making fantastic time, so much better than I had predicted. Based on my time at Ilfracombe Tri, which was 2:53:55, I had predicted six to six and a half hours for this event, as it's

EIGHT

twice the distance and with a tougher bike and run route … and the dreaded sea swim, of course.

Tears well up as I realise I'm going to achieve this in a better time than I could ever have dreamed of. So what if I'm not as quick as others – I'm almost 50 years old and probably two stone heavier than the other competitors.

Another thought pops into my head: I told the family not to expect me until 2pm earliest – at this rate they're going to miss me, as I will be in before they get there. I'm laughing and crying out loud … I know I can be an Ironman … I just know it!

Bike in, and out I go on to the run. It's a beautiful trail run alongside the river and waterfalls of Watersmeet. My legs are screaming with pain as I try to run; this is the worst bit of a triathlon, switching from bike legs to run legs. The paths are scattered with tree roots, stones, muddy puddles and tourists. There's plenty of encouragement along the way from Sunday morning strollers and dog-walkers.

Before I know it I'm on the final stretch from the trail run, and a team-mate has come out to meet me. Sarah Logan is my escort; she pushes me to keep my legs going, and as tourists meander along the streets, she's shouting out 'Runner coming through!' and clearing a path for me. I feel very, very special. A few yards left and I cross the finish line, knowing I've beaten my predicted time, but not knowing by how much.

As they put a medal around my neck, I glance up and see my family. They made it – just! They had only just arrived and were checking the screens for my times when my name was being announced. Wow, what a tough event! But wow, what a time. I predicted six hours – I actually finished in 5:00:20! Funnily enough, I also won a prize for being third in my age category! OK, so there were only three in the category, but I will milk this as it's unlikely I will ever win a prize again!

* * * * *

Everything is moving fast very suddenly. You can wish and dream for something, but when you do something to trigger it, it can then all happen faster than you can imagine. Just a few weeks ago, it was suggested to me that I could look for a sponsor. That triggered an email, which seemed positive on first response – but, having learned you never get what you really want, I wasn't going to be holding my breath.

Well, today it happened! A phone call from my potential sponsor, Nicola Dames at Vanilla Blush, in conjunction with Trio Ostomy Care, and she's said yes! Oh my word, it's really going to happen. Not only are they going to sponsor me, but they've done some initial research and don't believe a woman in Europe with an ostomy has ever tackled a full Ironman triathlon. This is even more valuable, as the media coverage could be pretty big in the ostomy world.

We're not just talking about putting their logos on my trisuit – Nicola is talking about creating a bespoke trisuit for this. And they don't want it revealed until nearer the day of Ironman – designed purely for that event. This is mind-blowing. My head is spinning at the pace things have happened. My determination has brought me to this point: my stubbornness to not let my ileostomy hold me back has given me a whole new lease of life.

I cannot describe how excited I am. We need to sort out the paperwork and then I can go and buy the bike. Buy the bike! That is surreal – my dream bike is actually going to be mine. I'm going to be competing in a serious

EIGHT

race on a serious bike! In fact, the bike's colours match one of my sponsors' colours beautifully. I think they will be very happy with this.

I know I will have to do some photography and video for them, but I am happy with that because it means I know I will be inspiring others who have an ostomy or who are having to confront stoma surgery. This could be a whole new turning point for me, fulfilling my personal desire to help others.

My training is going to be rigorous. I don't want to let my sponsors down or my family down. I don't want to 'just finish' at Ironman, I want to finish it with time in hand. This is just so exciting – this is real!

* * * * *

The next Sunday morning, I get up feeling just a little bit jaded after a night out with the girls. Throughout the season I have hardly touched any alcohol, so having just a couple of drinks can have quite an effect on me, but I still head for the pool for the tri club Sunday swim session. Coached sessions usually consist of mixed drills, and I now find myself heading to the intermediate lane, rather than the 'Lane One Lovelies'. But what bad timing ... today, of all days, our club coach decides we are going to do a 1,500m time trial. Yes: 60 lengths non-stop. After some warm-up drills, we're off – three lanes of triathletes ploughing up and down the pool. It must be quite a sight for onlookers.

My toes get touched a few times by the swimmer behind me, and I stop briefly at the end of the lane for them to pass me. Thank goodness my own training sessions are usually 2,000–3,000m: doing 1,500m doesn't seem so daunting.

I'm holding my own at a steady pace, and whilst I am slower than most, I do have the sheer fitness to swim endurance distance. My time is 39 minutes 52 seconds. Wow – I was expecting around 45 minutes, so this is fantastic. When I do the maths afterwards, this shows I am swimming throughout at pretty much my race pace. It doesn't seem all that long ago when I was just pleased to swim two lengths of the pool.

On long swims, I find that I 'zone out'; in fact, I find myself thinking of all sorts of things – what I've got in for dinner tonight, where I'm going later, those sorts of random thoughts. The physical activities of swimming – moving my arms and legs at the right time, and my breathing – are now so automatic that I hardly think about them.

The feedback from my colleagues, who haven't seen me swim for some time, is that I had a perfect form and one of them was 'blowing out of her arse' to catch me. What a fantastic phrase – I don't have an arse to blow out of! It feels great to know others can see my progress; when you train continuously and always time yourself against a clock, you never see the change. Just like watching the hands of a clock going round slowly but surely.

Tomorrow, as I don't have my training buddy with me, I am going to see how long it takes me to swim 4,000m – the Ironman distance – to set myself a benchmark. Just like I have been told about marathons, you shouldn't have to go the full distance before the day, just build up and peak on race day, but I want to see how I fare. I will be happy to swim for 2 hours, but my ultimate goal is to swim it in 1 hour 45 minutes. I know that's pushing my limits a bit, but if you don't push yourself you never improve.

EIGHT

After the joy of my swim success, my head turns to running. Recently, everyone has been telling me that they have not got a place in the Virgin London Marathon (VLM). I too had put my name in the ballot for a place (I know I am shooting above myself again), and it's starting to concern me that I haven't heard. Have I missed an email or piece of post? Then today my friend, who also hasn't heard, announces she's got a place. Does that mean they send out all the 'no' answers first? Does this mean I might have a place? I'm actually very nervous and excited all at once. The longer I wait, the more nervous and excited I am getting.

A little niggle in my head thinks perhaps I'm in, but I mustn't think like that, because if I get a 'no' I will be even more gutted. I need to focus on my run; I really struggle with it. I clearly need loads of work on this discipline. At the moment, I still have a run/walk strategy, but I need to do more running than walking. Oh well, yet another day of waiting. Everyone should be notified by 7 October, so only two more days of torture.

Two days later and my emotions are running rife. I know I'm almost 50 and going through the menopause, but this Ironman journey seems to be stretching my emotions to the limit. I don't believe it's tiredness, but the recognition of what I have done so far and what I intend to do next July.

Today is the latest date by which all Virgin London Marathon runners will be notified of whether they have a ballot place or not. I've still not had anything in the post or by email, and I'm on tenterhooks … and then we don't get any post this morning. I therefore ring the help desk and sit in a telephone queue for half an hour until someone picks up my call: 30 minutes of agonised waiting for a man to tell me within two minutes that I haven't got a place in the ballot.

I am gutted – more than I imagined I would be. I'd been hoping that the wait meant I'd got a place. After hearing so many people saying they got a place, I feel rather numb and actually disappointed that I haven't received the letter and I've had to resort to making a phone call to find out. The built-up emotion overwhelms me as I feel tears welling up, but I give myself a stiff talking-to; there are plenty more marathons I could do.

But, as one door closes, another one opens. A young woman who I've come to know through the Ostomy Lifestyle Athletes group has got a place in the ballot but has already run it twice before, and she has offered me her place. Part of me wants to grab it, but she deserves the slot for herself. After some honest conversation, she really does want me to run in her place. She's been seriously unwell and struggling with her stoma, and she's admitted she is not sure she would get round, that's if she even got to the start line. What a completely selfless and generous thing to do. I know I want the place for personal (even selfish) reasons, but now it's all the more important that I train and run this event to the best of my abilities, representing her and her faith in me.

She is such a wonderful person – someone who I've never even yet met face-to-face has sacrificed her place for my dreams. I owe her so much. Tears start to flow and just don't stop. This has been an emotional rollercoaster day. Now I've got to kick myself up the backside and get running. The marathon is in April.

Chapter Nine

IT'S A Tuesday in mid-October and I'm stuck in a hotel in Coventry – sadly not as good as it had looked on the website at the time of booking, so I've got time to ponder. I've not trained since Saturday, as I've had guests down at home, and I'm getting twitchy. As soon as I arrived in the hotel, I had to ask where I could run. It's too dark now in an area I don't know; but, sitting at a table for one waiting for dinner, I've found the nearest park, which looks like it's got some great paths for running. I cannot believe I'm actually looking forward to getting up early and going for a run. I think the appeal is because it's in a different area.

Yesterday afternoon, I helped out with the children's running club after school. We took 12 children under the age of ten for a two-mile run. It was absolutely lovely. We set a very gentle pace for them, and I loved it; I am truly beginning to love the running. I want to be able to run so much longer consistently. I've got until April to prepare for the Virgin London Marathon and still a long way to go.

I'm becoming a numbers person – how many lengths, how many metres, how many minutes per kilometre. The focus, for the triathlons, seems to have peaked right at the end of the season. Up until now I have just seen myself as a newbie – a mum who just about crosses the finish line in time. It's starting to creep into a bit of an obsession, but I must keep the balance of training right with the family. That's why my training always takes place early in the morning.

I can get out and ride or swim at 6am or 6.30am and be at my desk in the week by 9am, or be home around 10 to 10.30am after a three- or four-hour cycle ride at the weekends. My body clock now naturally wakes me up at 4.30 to 5am. This is *my* time! It's just a shame my body doesn't switch off once in a while to let me have a lie-in. I need to start going to bed earlier to get more rest. I cannot increase my training on just five hours' sleep per night.

So tonight, with a hotel room to myself, I am going to go to bed early, chill out with a cup of tea and get myself an early night. Then I should be bright and ready for a 10km run in the morning. After all, my training buddy, Al, went out tonight to up the target to 1:05:02. Let's see how close I can get to this.

* * * * *

With Trio Ostomy Care going ahead as one of my sponsors, alongside Vanilla Blush, things have moved fast. Despite not having the paperwork sorted yet, we need to make the most of the weather as Trio want to film an advertisement of me training, using their products. I have scouted out the area and found some spots that I think would give a good backdrop up across Exmoor.

After I met the film crew of three from Into Production for a quiet drink on Wednesday night, we're planning to film on Thursday and Friday. Just talking to them about

NINE

what they have in mind is exciting. They describe it as being a bit like a *Rocky* montage; I cannot quite picture it myself, but I'll trust it turns out all right. These three people are so easy to chat to. I get on with most people, but I guess it's part of their job to make the person who's going to be in front of the camera relaxed. They've filmed for Trio and Vanilla Blush before, so I've seen some of their work, which is amazing. I cannot believe I am going to be the focus of their video. Not only are we filming a video of my training and endeavours to be an Ironman, but they also need a night-time product video to demonstrate how confidently people can sleep with Trio Ostomy Care products, so we're going to be busy over the next two days.

Thursday – today we are going to be filming with me cycling across Exmoor and some running. For the run, I've chosen Watersmeet down in Lynmouth, because it's so stunning and, in a way, I want the video to show north Devon at its best. We head up on to the moors to start the day for the bike footage. I had found two locations and sent video clips in advance, which is exactly where they now choose to pull in to do the first shoot. The views are stunning across Exmoor, and there are lots of wild ponies grazing close by. We don't use the main road here, as it would be awkward with traffic, but a little sidetrack alongside the car park area gives us a great spot. If I thought I would be able to turn today into a bit of fartlek training, I'm wrong. I have to cycle a very short distance backwards and forwards until they like what they've got on film. It doesn't bother me, though – it's all rather fun.

Aaron, the cameraman, is squashed into the boot of their car with the hatchback open, with the camera on a tripod. They have to drive up and down whilst I follow them. I have to keep close to the back of the car, but they're not actually driving fast enough for me and I'm constantly having to put on my brakes so as not to run into them.

Now we're into some of the slow-motion detail shots – putting on a glove, clipping on my helmet, clicking my cleat into my pedal, and then a little braking to create a crunch/dust-up from my rear wheel. Everything has to be genuine for a road bike: there's no point in stopping with a big spray of gravel, as you just wouldn't do that – that's more a mountain bike thing.

We move on to another location on Exmoor, where we have a large car park to use as well as the road sweeping up through the hills. Now I have to ride up an incline as they want to film me working harder. More sitting behind the car required! This time I have to work to keep up with the car going up the incline, but on the descent I'm braking hard and have to tell them to speed up so I don't hit them. We have fun dreaming up some shots. They've got a GoPro camera, which sits on the end of a bendy arm. They want to put the GoPro on my handlebars. How naïve of me then, thinking they wanted to film the road in front: no – they want to film my face! Possibly luckily for me, the GoPro arm drifts downwards as I'm riding, but I don't notice, so they are probably filming the sky. Gaffer tape comes in handy to strap the arm on to the bottom of my drop bars, so we can film my chain shifting up and down the rings as I ride.

We're overrunning because Damian, the film director, is so excited at all the fabulous scenery that he wants to get as much as possible.

In the car park we have to shoot some drive-bys, filming alongside me. There's no one else parked up here, so we have a great spot across the car park with the valleys behind us as the backdrop. After two or three takes, a car

NINE

pulls in, and none of us can believe where they park: right in the middle of where we are filming! It's like going to a cinema which is almost empty and having someone sit down right in front of you, despite all the empty seats they could choose from. The lady is very accommodating when we ask if they would mind moving their car out of shot, and asks if we are filming an advert. As they start to reverse out of our way, another car pulls in and parks next to the space she is vacating. We cannot believe this: you can see we are driving horizontally across this section of the car park! I move up to the second car, and as the man starts to get out of the driver's seat I ask if he'd kindly reverse back across the car park so he is out of shot. He huffs and moans, 'Only want to use the bloody toilets!' I cannot believe his response; there's a whole car park and the toilets are on the other side, so why park where we are filming and then moan when he's asked to move?

Clarissa is my make-up lady and general helper. She touches up my make-up and makes me feel like a superstar; she's absolutely lovely. She's enamoured with my bike, and I let her have a go at riding it around the car park.

Time is moving on, and we head down to Watersmeet, where I had competed in Tri the Beast. We park up the hill, and we have to carry all the camera gear we're going to need, as it's a bit of a trek down to where the two valleys and rivers meet. Time for a change of clothes for me: now into trail shoes and running kit.

Watersmeet is stunning and thankfully quite quiet today. At the bottom of a deep gorge at the confluence of the East Lyn River and the Hoar Oak Water, the tranquillity of the place is surreal, with just the sound of the water tumbling over the rocks and wildlife in the surrounding woodland.

Damian's very excited at the location again. With the camera set up down at water level, I have to run backwards and forwards across the bridge over the meeting of the two rivers. Whilst they watch the footage back, I realise that this is exactly where I played in the water with my sisters, Sally and Amanda, when we were 14, 12 and 7 years old. My dad, Bob Olden, was sat mid-stream with us whilst my mum, Diana, took a photograph. That image springs to mind as I stand on the water's edge. I can see us stood here in the water. Having lost my dad to a heart attack when he was just 52, it seems very poignant to film in exactly this spot. It makes me feel like he's here with me, watching what I am doing, just as he did all those years ago. I am sure he would be proud, if not aghast that I'm a bit mad taking on such a challenge as Ironman.

It's my 50th birthday soon, and I am acutely aware that when my dad was 50 he didn't know that he had only two more years to live. Did he feel as young as I do? Whilst your body grows older, your mind doesn't. There's so much I still want to do in my life, and I believe I've got many years to grow old. I have no doubt that my dad thought the same too. He was still working when he died suddenly, and I now appreciate how he was cut down in his prime.

I'm also conscious that, only two years short of the age he was when he passed away, I am putting my body through intense pressure. Do I have the same issue as my dad? Is it genetic that his heart failed and mine will too? Have I got only two years left? My children are so young, I'd hate to leave them now. Maybe I'm being just a bit

NINE

paranoid, especially being aware of any twinges I feel in my chest when I'm training.

I need peace of mind that my heart is strong and I can do this. Thousands of people take part in Ironman triathlons, but there are occasional deaths from putting your body under such intense strain. I must build up my strength gradually so my body can cope; my muscles will build, but I want to be sure my heart is strong.

I'm going to see my GP and ask her to check me over. I know this sounds a bit over the top, but then they always put warnings on anything strenuous, or even diets, to check with your GP that you are fit to take part.

Just a few close-ups at Watersmeet left to do. There's a steep set of steps cut into the ground alongside the water, and Aaron sets up the camera to film my feet running up them. 'Action!' I hear him shout. I run up the steps. 'Cut! I'm sorry, Caroline, I missed them. I didn't realise how quick you'd run up them.' We all laugh at him. He has to pan the camera up and thought it would be slow!

We drive back to the Barnstaple Hotel, where they are staying, as we need to shoot some footage for the second video, which demonstrates how you get a good night's sleep wearing the Silex flange extenders. Yesterday I checked with reception that we might be able to use a bedroom for filming, and we were told that it would be no bother. Today, it's a different girl on reception, and she asks the manager – neither of them has been notified. He's a bit wary: filming? In a bedroom? To be honest, it does sound a bit dodgy, especially when there are four of us!

The best he can do is ring and leave a message on his director's mobile number. So much for him having responsibility for the hotel. We are running out of time and head up to Aaron's bedroom, where we discuss whether the issue with the hotel is a) they don't have a spare room for us to use or b) they're not comfortable about us filming some bedroom scenes. We reckon it's the latter. After a quick phone call to the director's PA, we get the all-clear to film.

We use Aaron's bedroom and turn it into a film set with lights and cameras. We film in reverse, seeing as I am still fully dressed in my daytime running kit. First, sit on the bed, lean forward, tie shoes, lean forward again, look out of the window wistfully, then walk out of shot. How many times we shot that, I just don't know – I lost count. They must have loads of close-ups of my feet. Then we do the bathroom scene. The bathroom is really small, so, whilst I stand at the sink, Aaron has his camera set up in the doorway and has to film into the mirror. The guys are really sweet and ask if I'm comfortable doing these shots, as I have to bare my stomach and have my stoma bag on display; they've worked with ostomates before and are very aware of how self-conscious we can be about our stomas. I can understand that if I were taking the stoma bag off completely – I'm not sure I'd be particularly confident about that. It's odd: I'm not at all shy about telling people about my stoma, but would I ever let anyone see it? Craig has always seemed a bit squeamish around it, but Robert and Natasha seem to have adopted it; it's like it's a pet, and they are always asking how 'strawberry' is if they happen to come in the bathroom when I am changing my bag.

It's my children who made me feel so accepting of my stoma when I first had my surgery. Having to change my bag at home is one thing, but going out in public and having to sort it out was a whole new ball game. When I first had my surgery, my children were only aged seven and five, so out shopping we'd all have to cram into the larger disabled cubicle. Their fascination with strawberry was so innocent and unreserved, it made it seem 'normal' to me having it. They gave me confidence to not be embarrassed about it. Yes, it can be smelly when emptying my bag, and people in the next cubicle might hear me 'rustling' around with my pouch, but so what? Some ladies fart loudly in public loos – really, they do!

Back to the filming: I don't have any concern about doing it, because I'm not taking my pouch off, just demonstrating how to put on the Silex flange extenders. So I have to show off my stomach with my bulgy bit where my stoma is ... so what, that's just me and there's no getting away from it. Sure, I'd love to have a flat stomach to wear the clingy dresses that still hang in my wardrobe. I know that if I train well I can have a much flatter stomach and my stoma won't be so prominent. Plus, now that Vanilla Blush are sponsoring me, their products are so sexy, beautiful and practical with a range of supportwear too, I can hide this multitude of sin ... whether I have a stoma or not.

Now we move to the 'bedroom scene'. I'm in my pyjamas, and I will be honest: I am more nervous about this. How daft! If we'd been in a room that wasn't that of one of the crew, I'd be fine; but, knowing that I am going to be 'sleeping' in Aaron's bed, which he slept in last night and will sleep in again tonight – that just feels odd!

After my initial nervousness at clambering in and out of his bed, it actually becomes fun. We've done the 'getting into bed' bit, now it's the 'go to sleep' bit. There have to be some practice runs, working out how I'm going to turn and switch the bedside light off without a full camera shot of my backside, and co-ordinating with the team to turn off all the set lights at the same time so it looks as though it goes dark. The curtains are drawn, but it's still light outside.

I have to turn over, shuffle, snuggle down a few times, then lay still for several minutes – this is being shot in time-lapse, so I have to 'sleep' for ten minutes for the camera. The room goes quiet; I'm actually relaxing into this. The crew whisper to each other. We only require the visual footage and there's no sound recording needed.

'You can talk loudly, you know. I'm not really asleep,' I call out from under the duvet, where my mouth cannot be seen by the camera. That breaks the quiet atmosphere. Trying not to giggle is hard, and listening to instructions with my eyes permanently shut feels weird. As 'daylight' comes up, I stir and actually wish I could stay in this bed. Day one of filming is complete.

Day two is at the beautiful Saunton Sands Hotel in Braunton. The hotel is exclusively booked out for a conference, but we have permission to film in their outdoor pool. We have to remember it's October, and whilst the sunshine gives the feel of summer, the air temperature is much cooler. After checking out the venue, we start with filming on Saunton beach whilst the tide is in, otherwise it's a long walk out to the sea. The plan is to film me walking out of the sea as though I've finished a swim, peeling off my wetsuit. We do this numerous times, but every time I have to put the top half of my wetsuit back on, it keeps getting 'stuck' on my arms – usually you'd only put your wetsuit on when you are dry, before a swim. Plus my hands are becoming so cold I cannot grip the wetsuit to pull it up. In fits of giggles, Clarissa – the film crew's runner and make-up artist – has to do it for me.

Damian, the film director, wants more footage in the sea, so he has to walk out knee-deep in his shorts with the

NINE

camera (which we absolutely must not get wet). Walking in and out of the waves, making sure to get plenty of splashing, I'm starting to get really cold. We get what we need, but Damian gets more than he bargained for when a wave smacks him between the legs. Payback!

Back at the hotel, our next 'set' is the outdoor pool. The guys have the main camera set up on the jib so they can swing it down and above the water level, and we're going to need the GoPro for shots actually in the water. What we need first, however, are robes to keep me warm – and Damian too, as he's drawn the short straw and is going to have to get in the pool too at some point for the underwater shots.

I'm only in a trisuit now, no wetsuit to keep me warm, and the pool is not heated – in fact, I wouldn't be surprised if they'd filled it with ice cubes before we arrived. It's freezing cold! We were warned it wouldn't be heated.

Step by step I go a little deeper into the pool; the cold takes my breath away. From the side, Damian calls out:

'Are you ready to go?'

'N...n...n...n...no,' I call back. 'I can't...g...g... get...m...my...br...br...breath yet!' I stutter through gritted teeth.

A minute or two later and I've acclimatised to the cold pool and swim a couple of lengths. My fingers are tingling, and I've got what my children would call 'brain freeze'. A few more lengths and I'm ready for them to film. As soon as they have what they need, I'm out of the water like a shot and wrapped up in a robe to warm up. Aaron takes the camera off the jib, sets it up poolside and films me doing some more lengths. But now they need some underwater footage. Hee hee – this is going to be fun! Damian has to get in the pool with the GoPro. As he steps in, he shrieks like a girl. Every step deeper, he squeals. The rest of us cannot stop laughing at his reaction to the cold water. This is real dedication to the task. It's hilarious.

'Everything I own has gone inside,' he claims through chattering teeth! I really am on the point of peeing myself laughing – at least that might have warmed the pool up! Damian sets the GoPro on the bottom of the pool with his foot, so he doesn't have to put his shoulders under the water. I swim over the top of the camera a number of times, and although I offer to dive down and retrieve the camera when we are finished, Damian braves it and ducks down to grab it, almost shrieking again at the cold. Sorry (not sorry), but I am in fits of laughter again. A bit of flyby filming underwater is needed and then we're done. I am so cold, Clarissa says my lips have gone blue!

All that's left now is some running on the beach as the sun goes down, but sadly today has been overcast, so we're unlikely to get the stunning orange sunset dipping into the sea that we've been seeing recently. Another change of clothes and a warm-up required. After the pool swim, I am chilled to the bone. Even though I have several layers of clothes on in the hotel, my core is still trembling – that was so darn cold! But at least I coped better than Damian. Cold exposure isn't such a bad thing, considering I have to swim in Lake Padarn at Snowdon in May. And I know that is cold, but at least I will have a wetsuit on then.

The beach runs are very short: just backwards and forwards in front of the camera for some more close-up foot action and a few final runs down the Braunton Burrows and across Saunton Sands as the light drops. It's a wrap!

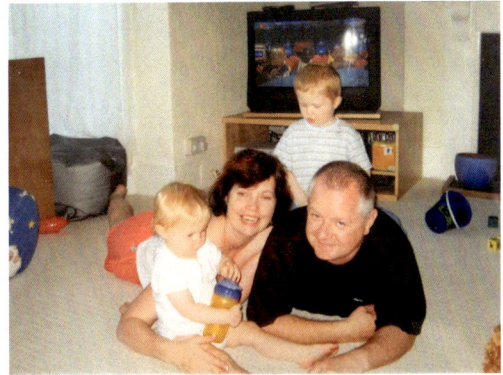

Family life as ulcerative colitis kicked in. (Left to right) Natasha, Caroline, Robert and Craig Bramwell.
Credit: Diana Olden

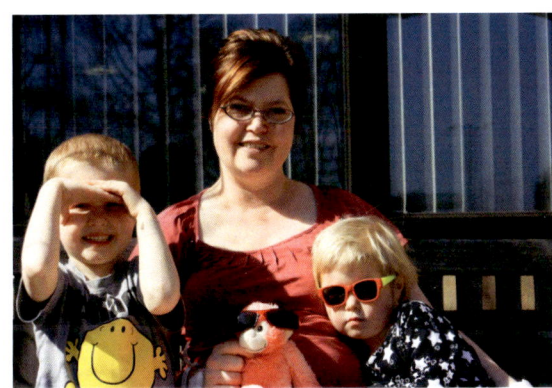

Surgery day.
Credit: Craig Bramwell

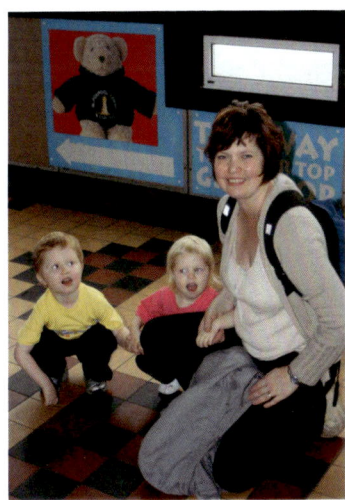

Steroids started to have the 'moon face' side effect.
Credit: Craig Bramwell

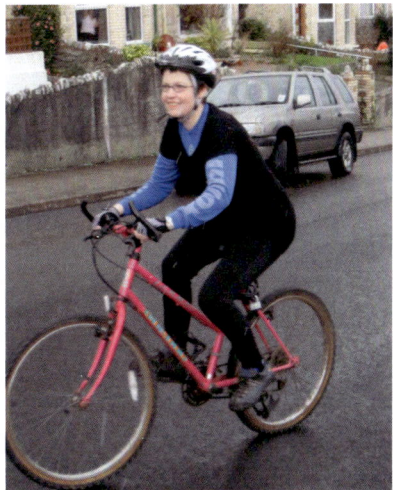

First day of training for London to Paris 24.
Credit: Craig Bramwell

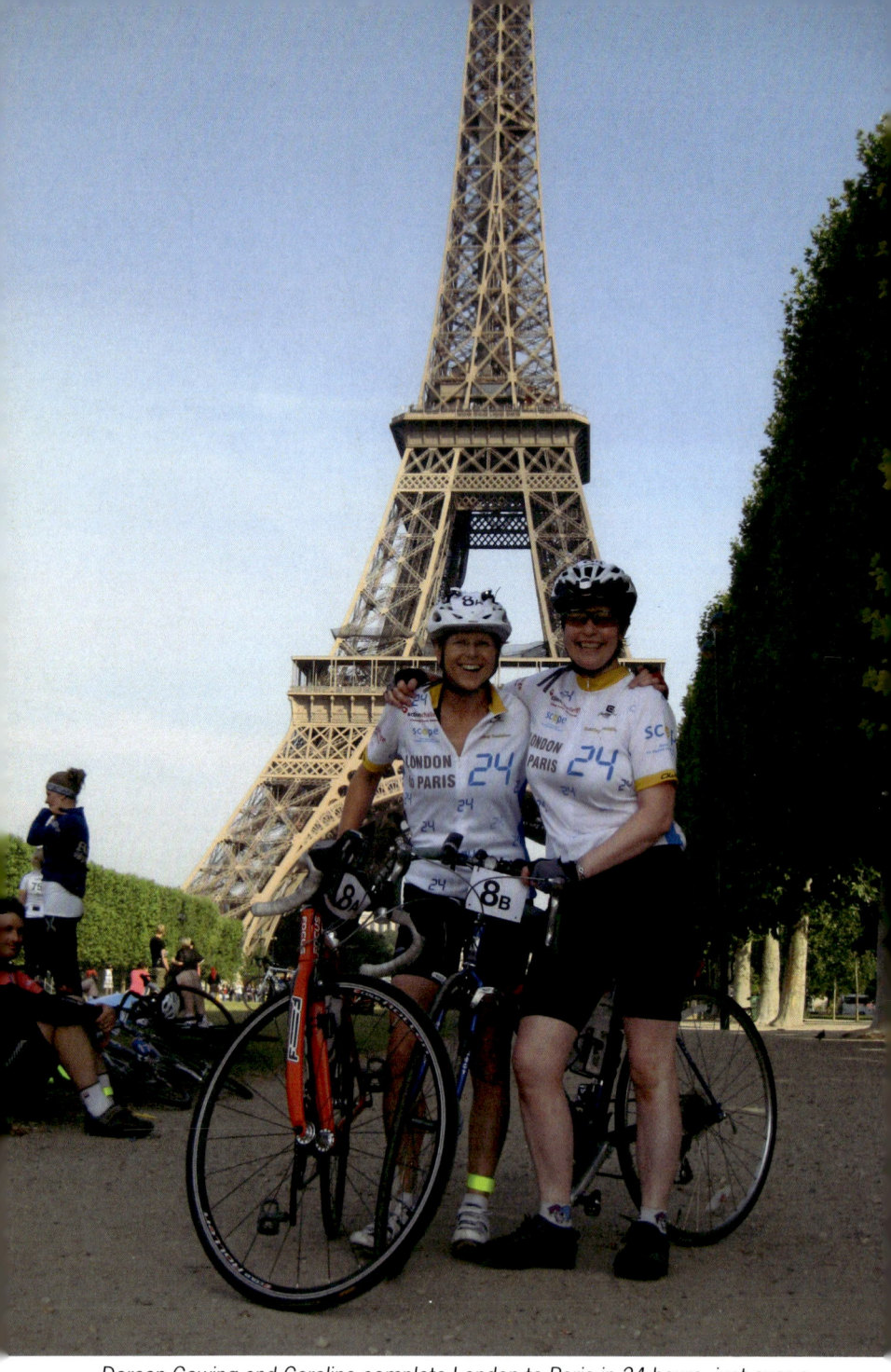

Doreen Gowing and Caroline complete London to Paris in 24 hours, just over a year after her surgery.

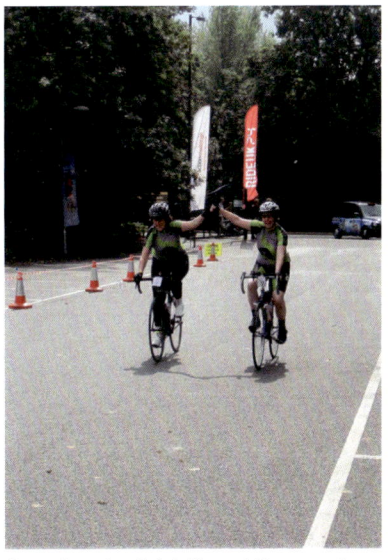

Crossing the finish line of Newcastle to London in 24 hours with Lucie Gallen.
Credit: Craig Bramwell

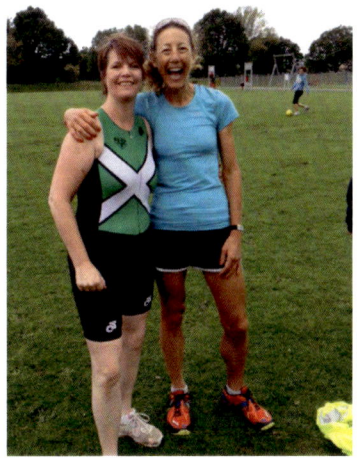

Caroline is inspired by four-time Ironman world champion, Chrissie Wellington, at Barnstaple Park Run.

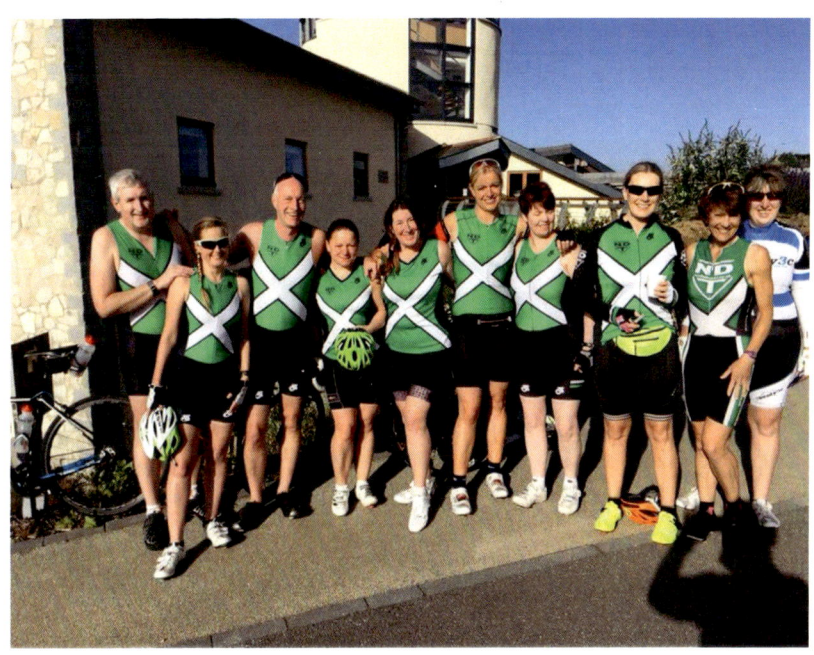

North Devon Tri members line up for Ride for Precious Lives.

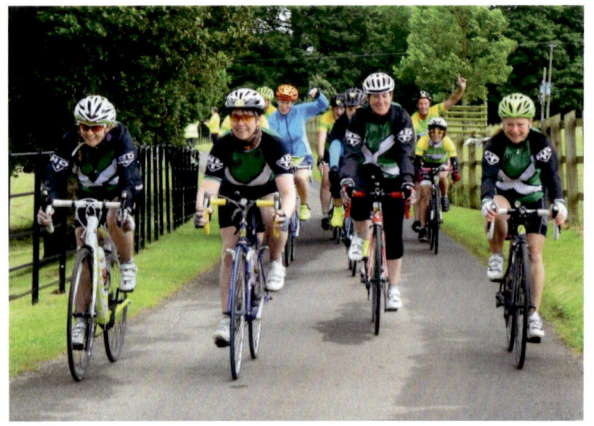

Crossing the line at Ride for Precious Lives. (Left to right) Sarah Logan, Caroline Bramwell, Elizabeth Mason, Graham Salisbury, Lucie Gallen, Tina Kiff-Jamieson, Mark Rhead, Susan Standford, Donna Marriott.

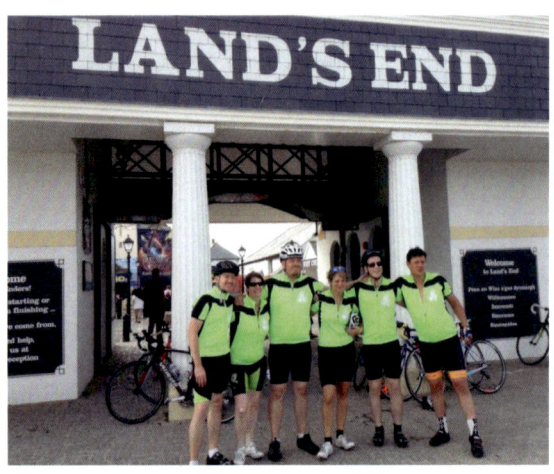

*Reaching Land's End.
(Left to right) Ed Johns, Caroline Bramwell, Darrel Gill, Jayne Jarrett, Peter Quincey, Olly Keates.*
Credit: Chrissie Trow

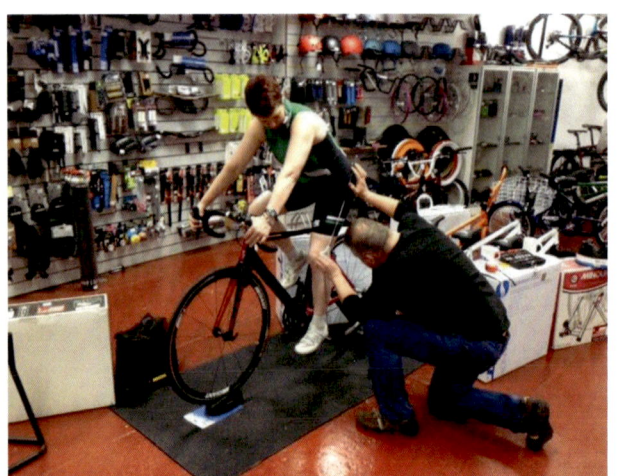

Caroline having her first ever bike fit with Lance Richmond at Bike It.

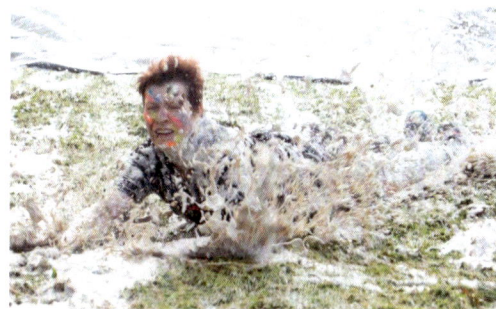

Taking part in Mission Unbreakable was brilliant fun – what stoma bag?
Credit: Andy Casey Photography

Competing in Tri the Beast at Lynmouth brought back memories of family holidays at Lynmouth. (Left to right) Caroline with Dad, Bob Olden, and sisters, Sally and Amanda.
Credit: Diana Olden

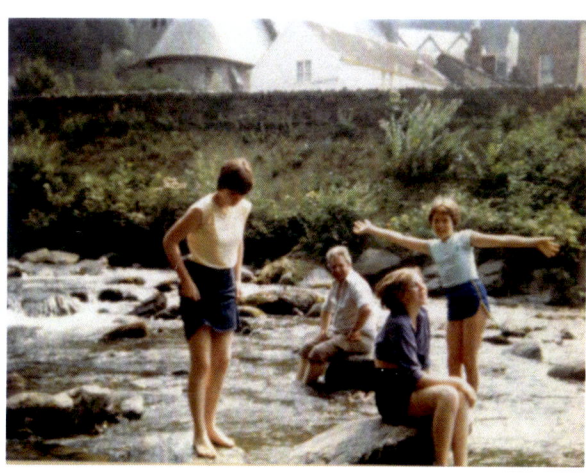

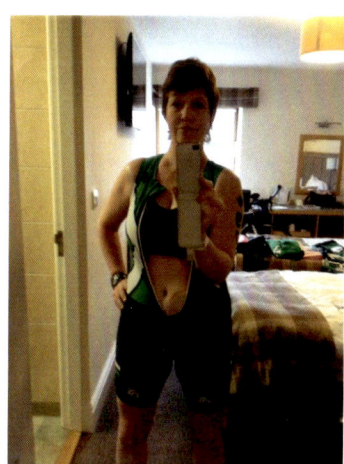

Having an ostomy bag wouldn't stop Caroline competing in Snowdonia Slateman Savage.

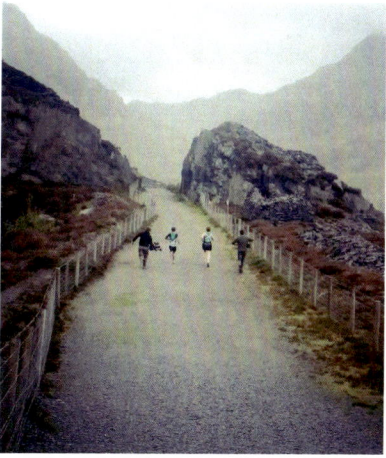

Filming at Snowdonia Slateman Savage for Trio Ostomy Care. (Left to right) Damian Cox, Samera Ismael, Caroline Bramwell, Aaron Hussein.
Credit: Into Productions

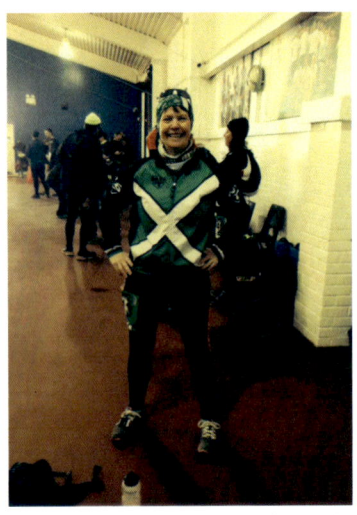

All togged up for Portland Coastal Half Marathon, ready to be battered by Storm Imogen.

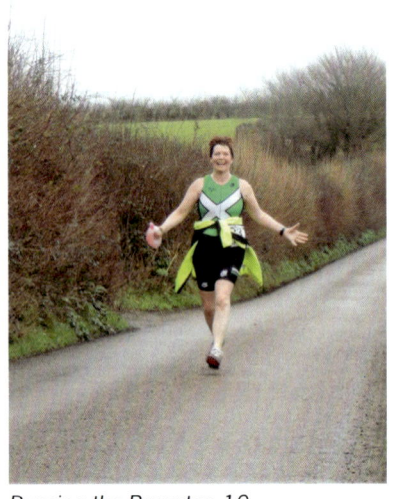

Running the Braunton 10. **Credit: Brian Mulholland**

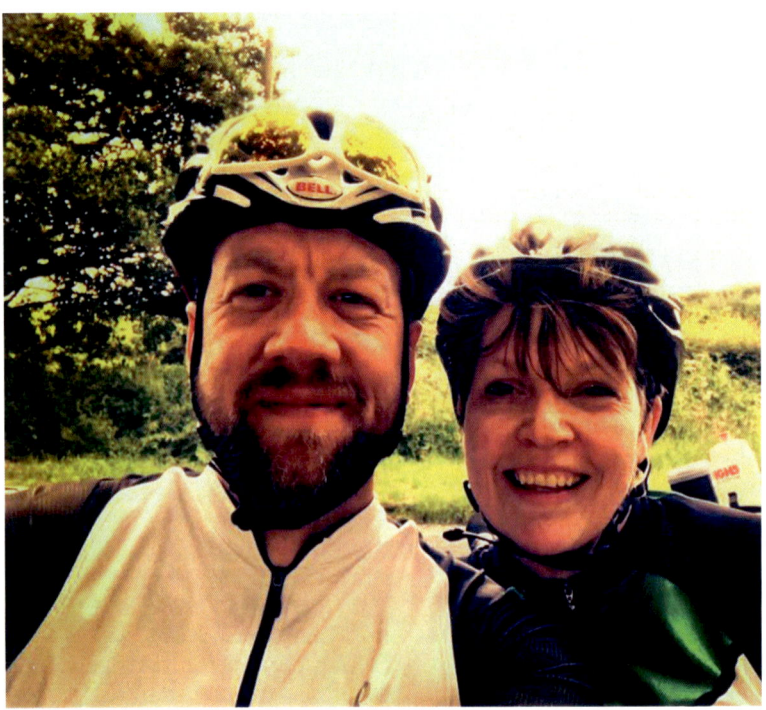

Fellow ostomate, Marc Mahoney, leads Caroline out on the Ironman course as part of training. **Credit: Marc Mahoney**

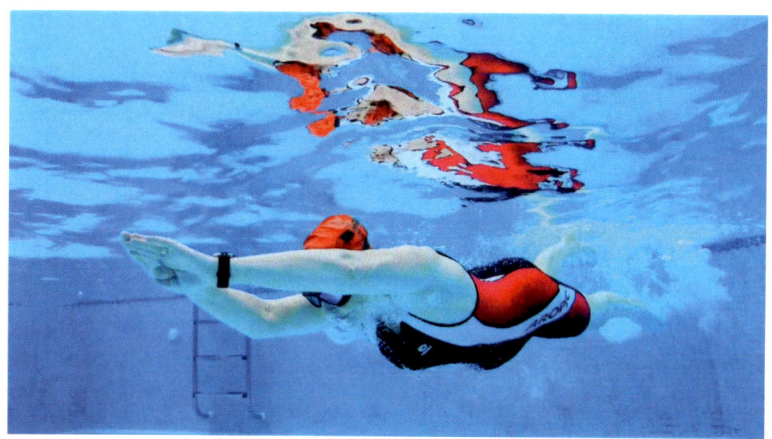

No longer afraid of being under water. **Credit: Into Productions**

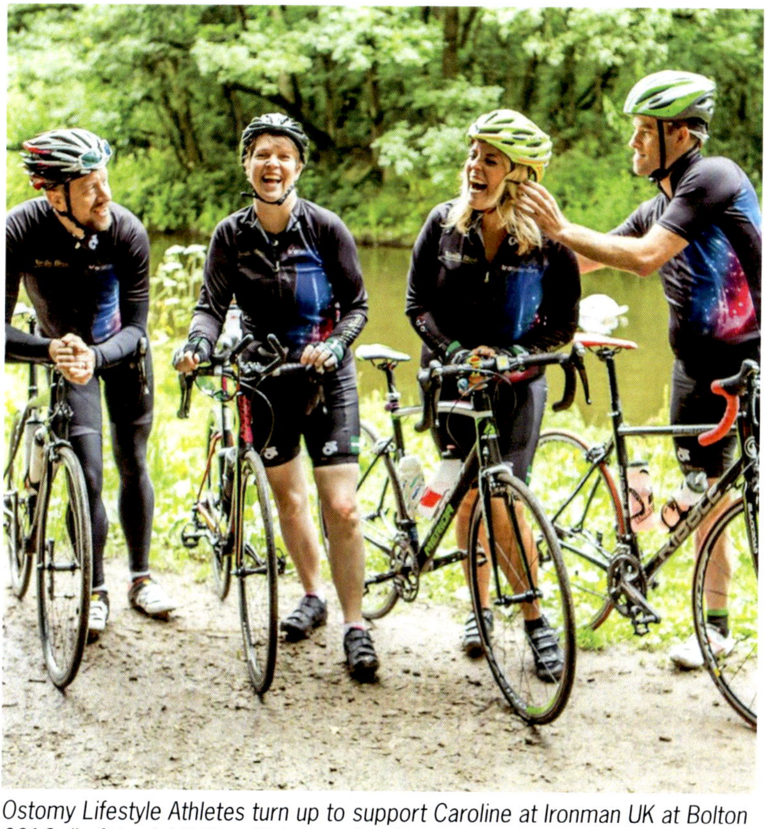

Ostomy Lifestyle Athletes turn up to support Caroline at Ironman UK at Bolton 2016. (Left to right) Marc Mahoney, Caroline Bramwell, Nicola Dames of sponsor Vanilla Blush, Mark Vos. **Credit: Into Productions**

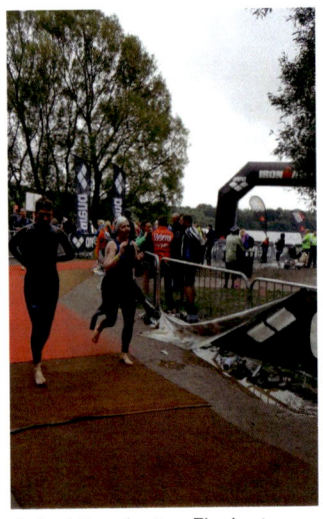

Out of Pennington Flash at Ironman UK 2016.
Credit: Tina Kiff-Jamieson

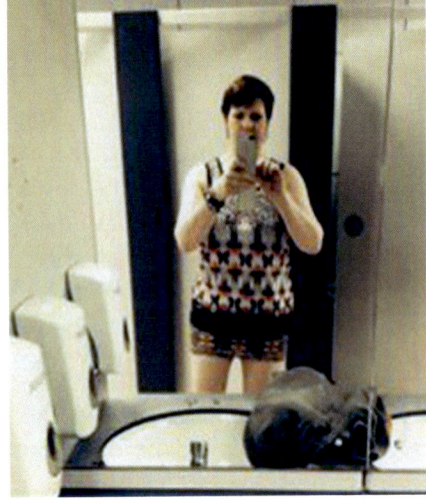

A sharp reminder that an ostomy can still kick back. Caroline improvises a new look.

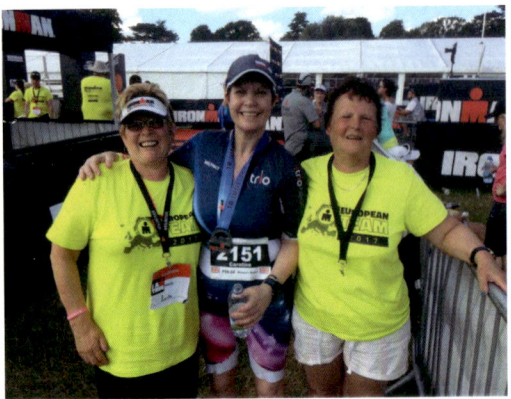

Volunteer 'Ironmums' Linda Ogden (left) and Janet Gibson (right) are always ready to support all the competitors.
Credit: Brian Mulholland

Trained and supported by Tri Force Endurance coaches, Billy Harris (left) and Simon de Burgh (right).
Credit: Brian Mulholland

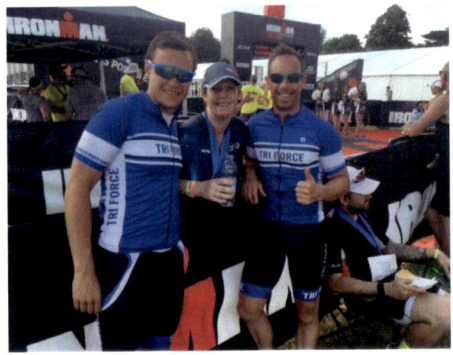

Chapter Ten

IT'S NOVEMBER and well past the end of the triathlon season, and plans are in place for training to be an Ironman next July. But I have been bitten by the bug and cannot just sit at home. So, to round off the year I have signed up for a 10km Mission Unbreakable commando-style event with Al, and today's the day to get out there.

You would assume that because you're constantly training, this wouldn't be too difficult. How wrong to make that assumption! In fact, it showed up my weaknesses, which, it turns out, means every muscle in my torso. Of course, I didn't know this on the day, but wow, did I know it the next day!

Commando obstacle courses are best done as a team – you need to motivate one another and help each other to overcome obstacles both physically and mentally. We, however, have dwindled to a team of just two! What we are to encounter and how we might overcome them is yet to be seen. In preparation for the unknown, I make the point of talking to other competitors at registration who have similar numbers written on their arms. Now I know that if we two get stuck, we'll have some backup on the course!

Fifteen minutes before we are due to start, we get put through our warm-up paces. Even this on its own immediately shows up my very obvious weaknesses. Running on the spot and being shouted at by a commando is fine, but I cannot do a single press-up. After my feeble attempts, we hold ourselves in position and then are told to roll (fast) along the ground, first one way, then back the other way. Seems great fun, but before long we're all dizzy and already we're covered in mud from rolling around on the wet ground.

No stopping now; without losing pace, Al and I jog over to the start line and we're off. This should be fun. A gentle jog across the field and we face our first challenge – a climbing net; we climb to the top, then up and over. One lady ahead of me was impressed with herself, as this was her biggest fear: heights. So, even on obstacle one she has achieved her aim. After scrambling over a wire fence, we have to pigeon-toe through a series of car tyres – not just once, but three times. I can see how they designed this as a way of warming up the legs.

A run through smoke takes us to the next field, where the first of our water challenges awaits us. We jump down into the cold water and wade along knee-deep. But it gets deeper and deeper. Not knowing how deep this is going to get is a little concerning, as the water level creeps up my things to my waist. Thankfully, I made sure I had put on a new stoma bag and flange extenders this morning, as I knew there would be water involved, but not how much. When the water gets to chest-high, it takes your breath away, but we both make it without getting dunked! Before us is a hill – a big, steep hill! We run (well, walk really) to the top, go around the post whilst drawing camouflage colours on our faces, then go back to the bottom. Twice

TEN

more we do this, on different parts of the hill with increasing steepness, painting our faces more and more as we go. This really does sap your legs of energy.

Just when you think your legs are heavy enough, we plunge headlong into a marsh – and I mean a real marsh, with big tall reeds and deep mud – up-to-your-knees mud. We try hopping from reed clod to reed clod, but there is no way we are going to avoid the suction pit of mud. With our feet sinking, cold mud sucks up our legs, and as we try to pull our feet out it's lucky we don't lose a shoe. One poor lady got so stuck in the mud and couldn't move, it took two men to pull her out as they ran by.

We run from field to field, feet leaden with mud, until we get washed down in another river. More swamps lead to mud crawls under barbed wire. We have to get down on our bellies and crawl through the sludge. Every reach of the arm leaves us elbow-deep in dark, stinking slime – and when a girl is just so filthy, with her hands plastered, there's only one thing she can do – throw it! Yes, throw it at her partner crawling along behind her, so a mud fight between Al and me ensues. I'm sure the commandos don't get to have this much fun.

I don't think I'd have ever had this much fun even without my bag. To be honest, crawling around on my tummy was one thing I never could do before my surgery. All those times when Robert and Natasha were small, playing in the lounge, and I couldn't even get down on the carpet to join them without risking a sudden urgent dash to the toilet. That was a different me, a me that I no longer recognise; this is the new, re-engineered me.

The final hurdles for us still lay ahead. My personal fear is the pull-through underwater. As we reach the water with a solid block of wood across it, there is a commando on either side. Between them is a single rope with knots tied in it, which disappears under the water. From the edge of the water, watching others go through, I can see that it is only a short distance, but once I am standing beside the commando in the water it looks endless. I'm panicking. I've no goggles, so all I am going to be able to do is shut my eyes, hold my breath and trust these two commandos with my life. This really is terrifying, even after all the swimming I do in the pool – this is way outside my comfort zone, and I'm considering bottling out.

Al goes through first and is waiting on the other side, encouraging me to be brave. The commandos are not going to force me to do anything I don't want to do. This one obstacle could beat me. I take a few more minutes to compose myself. Fear and panic will make me worse. I need to focus and relax. Everyone else has been under here, and everyone has come out the other side safely. There's only so much reasoning you can do with yourself. I am going to have to either get out and let it beat me, or commit wholeheartedly to it.

I grab the knotted rope, give a nod to the commando and – on the count of three – push myself under. With no vision, it is still terrifying; it feels as though I am floating up under the wooden board and I might get stuck under there. My grip on the rope is rock-solid, and I feel the yanking on the other end. Within seconds, which felt so much longer, I am up on the other side, trembling and spluttering, but I made it. I did it. This course can throw what it likes at me. I won't be beaten.

After lugging some tree trunks around, and running up more hills, the fun bit is next. The super slide. The big kids in all of us come out to play, as the plastic sheeting going all the way down a long hill, with straw bales on

TEN

either side and a tanker-ful of soapy solution, turns this into the best-ever bubble slide. Flat on my belly, oblivious to my stoma, I throw myself down the slippery slope. Clothes filled with soap bubbles, we run like two fluffy snowmen to the final obstacle. The ice bath is a skip full of freezing cold water. On the roadside, the locals have all come out to watch the competitors climbing up the breeze blocks to get into the skip, and to watch with glee the way they all have to manhandle each other in the cold water to get out the other side.

After crossing the final field, we run across the finish line. We may have only been a team of two, but we had our chance to race together.

* * * * *

Over recent weeks, I've got used to the idea of having a sponsor for my Ironman journey, but it has all been verbal. However, today the contracts arrived in the post. I have two co-sponsors, Vanilla Blush and Trio Ostomy Care. It's great to be representing these brands, and I've had some lovely conversations with Nicola from Vanilla Blush and Reena Patel at Trio, but as yet have not met either of them face-to-face. In my mind, having the contract agreements was more a formality, but actually picking up my pen to sign them, I get a surge of excitement and nervousness. I am not sure exactly how to describe it: it's a sense of responsibility. I love the products of both of these companies, and now I am an official representative of their brands. They have entrusted me to do my best both for myself and for them.

Aiming high to be an Ironman is a dream I know can come true, but now I want to do it even more and even faster. There's a 17-hour cut-off in an Ironman triathlon, with strict discipline cut-offs inside that time. The swim is 2.4 miles, which has to be completed within 2 hours 20 minutes of your start time. The 112-mile bike course then has two cut-offs within it, one at around 60 miles and another around 80 miles. If you don't get to either of these mileage points by a set time, you get cut straight away. You cannot keep riding to the second transition. If you do make it to the run, you then have a marathon in front of you, and you must finish the race before the final cut-off of 17 hours. Even if you cross the line a few seconds after this, you are not an Ironman. It's harsh, but if you didn't have to chase the clock, anyone could do it over any length of time. The challenge is not only to complete the three disciplines, but finish them in a set time.

I don't want to just scrape through at Ironman UK – I want to come through with time in hand. I want Vanilla Blush and Trio Ostomy Care to see that they have my total commitment, and their trust in me has pushed me even further.

* * * * *

It's nearly Christmas, and I cannot believe how fast the last six weeks have gone by. Since signing my sponsors' contracts, so much has kicked into play. I reckon it's the excitement within me that has rolled from week to week so fast. There's a lot to do between now and Ironman UK in Bolton, but at the rate the weeks are currently flying by, it will be here before I know it. I am excited for the day and the challenge, but it is just one day. The excitement is in the journey, reaching little goals along the way that show me I am improving.

So, since the contract, I have received my sponsorship funding and gone on the best shopping trip ever. OK, to

TEN

non-athletes, buying a bike is probably no different to buying a new washing machine – but to me this is like buying a super-turbo engine for my race. Lance and Luke at Bike It in Barnstaple have been a great help. In fact, they seem to have been infected with my excitement – they really want to do the best to help me achieve my dream.

That beautiful Giant Envie that I had looked at several months ago is now mine; she's black and pink with orange inside the front forks. I name her 'Piston'. I know it seems daft to give a bike a name, but this bike will have a personality; she will get me through the toughest things I have ever done. Why Piston? Well, it was the mantra I learned from Doreen back when I trained for London to Paris: 'My legs are pistons.' This bike is my extra piston.

Knowing I have the budget, I have decided to use the sponsorship money on the bike with a drink system and aero bars, new shoes and a smart Kask crash helmet. Also on my shopping list are some new running shoes and a coach. It was a dilemma whether I go for the carbon wheels or a coach, but the reality is that just being on this bike will make me faster, so the slight improvement with carbon wheels wouldn't really be noticed at my level of riding. However, having a coach to train me properly will have a much greater impact on my final results. Plus, a coach will motivate me far more than two wheels will. Who knows, next year I might find another sponsor and upgrade again. Listen to me – talking about 2017 when I haven't even reached 2016 yet.

A week later, it is bike fit day, and this is actually the first time I have properly sat on my bike. As I walk into Bike It, she is set up on the turbo ready for me. I feel like a kid at Christmas, itching to play with her new toys. I've had to wear my trisuit for this, as I am learning all the minutiae from Lance, the guy who's doing the bike fit for me, about how the professionals set up, when even the thickness of pad inside your trisuit can alter your saddle position by a couple of millimetres. This isn't like your old-fashioned bike set-up that you had when you got a new bike as a kid, this is a serious set-up.

This may seem all a bit over the top for a novice like me, and Craig keeps reminding me: 'You're not an elite rider'; but he doesn't seem to realise that if you want to perform well, you have to train like the professionals. After all, that's how I became a triathlete in the first place: 'If I want to be a triathlete, I have to train with triathletes.' Maybe I just talk about it a little too much at home.

I am a big believer that if you want something hard enough, then you have to surround yourself with like-minded people and those who you admire and aspire to be. If you always think 'I'll never be able to do that,' then guess what – you're right, you never will. It's all about having a positive mental attitude, not just in sport, but in any aspect of your life – I think I am naturally a bit crazy, prone to doing things on a whim, but I enjoy life like that! Not so long ago, I couldn't even leave my house, so just having the opportunity to do crazy things is a godsend. People who tell me I cannot do something or tell me I'm not good enough are not the kind of people I want around me. Having this crazy 'I can do anything' attitude can also be a positive help to others; I'm not afraid to push boundaries. I think that's why I have received so much support and encouragement from others. I've even had a lady in our North Devon Tri Club (most of whom now know about my stoma) tell me that I am a hero to many of them. I can honestly say this brought a tear to my eye. These triathletes are all amazing, and it is great to be able

TEN

to train and compete with them, albeit a lot further down the pack. They are like a second family now.

Back to the bike fit: nearly two hours of hopping on and off the bike, adjusting the seat post, shifting the saddle and measuring the angles on my legs and arms to make sure I have the optimum position for maximum power output. The bike feels so smooth and so quiet; it's actually the fact it's so quiet that surprises me the most. I'm so accustomed to the clicks and clunks of my old Peugeot Audax that this one seems heavenly. But then, I am taking a huge leap with this bike. It's a shame, therefore, that the weather now is so bad that I cannot take her out for a spin.

Two days later and there's a glimmer of sunshine – I cannot resist it, I manage to take my beautiful new bike out for her maiden ride of a little 10km. It's still windy, and, being on this new light bike, I feel every gust. I've had the aero bars fitted, which are a whole new experience, and I'm nervous about getting down on these before I've tried them out on the turbo trainer, and on a day when there's no wind. Looks like I will not be doing this until springtime, then.

My next investment is my coach. Wow, this is getting serious. Having someone who has experienced GB qualification triathlons and knows what it takes for me to become an Ironman will make a big difference. There are plenty of books on training for an Ironman triathlon, and I've already invested in a few of them. However, for me, I recognise that I need that kick up the backside – I need to be accountable to someone for training. Having a book with a set training plan is great and works for many people, but let's be honest here, I can be lazy and life can get in the way. Having a husband and two young children with various school commitments and after-school clubs will always come first. It's easy to say, 'I didn't have time to run today, I'll do it tomorrow.' But, of course, tomorrow comes around and I feel I should be doing something else. A sporadic training programme like this might not get me to the cut-offs, let alone to the finish line. So my search for a coach begins, but it doesn't take me long, as James Lapish is involved with our North Devon Tri Club and he's already competed at GB qualifier level himself.

We arrange to meet for a chat over coffee, after I have only told him the basics of my situation – a mum of two young children, married, running two businesses and publishing a magazine. Add to that the fact that I've got a stoma, which means my digestion system doesn't work quite like other athletes; with no large intestine, I only have around 80 per cent absorption and will dehydrate much quicker.

I am therefore very impressed when we meet, as not only has he read up on my condition, he's also found other extreme athletes who have had similar issues, who he can turn to for guidance. He's particularly keen to ensure my nutrition and hydration are spot-on, as, without a large intestine, my body cannot absorb as much calorie content or fluids, so this is going to be key to my training. It's also great to hear his excitement about my endeavour to be an Ironman, as I'm not your run-of-the-mill athlete. There's more to learn and work together on – something to 'get my teeth into' as he says. I reckon we're going to work really well together, learning and developing along the way.

Being a user of social media to share news about how I'm doing, I excitedly post up on Facebook that I have hired myself a new coach to get me ready for Ironman UK. Loads of friends congratulate me on hiring James,

TEN

who many of them know, but there is one remark on there which really gets to me in a bad way. I don't spot the remark at first as I'm not at my computer, but I get a couple of private messages on my mobile phone saying, 'Glad to hear you know what type of coach you need. Positive choices.' How odd, I think. What on earth does that mean?

It's only when I see the comment on my post that I truly understand the private message. The comment was from the man who had, a year ago, offered to help me with my triathlons. He used to be part of the Tri Club but left them many years ago. A year ago, knowing I needed guidance, I welcomed the generous offer of him 'coaching' me for free. I would join his small posse of triathletes for swimming sessions both at the pool and in the sea. I have a big fear of the sea, so even putting my face in the water in the sea (when I can do it in a pool) was a big issue for me.

He didn't charge to help me – it was more of a group of triathletes of various levels – although most of them were guys and were way above my level, and his approach to triathlon training was to 'be selfish'. Now I know that triathlon can be a selfish sport, but having a husband, young family and business to juggle, I couldn't just ignore them and be so pig-headedly selfish towards training. Plus I'm not a professional triathlete and nor do I expect to be one; I just want to finish the events I enter, to continuously improve. So I could see there were going to be a few issues here if this 'coach' didn't understand what my training meant and how it had to fit in with my lifestyle. In fact, when I told him that I had signed up to take part in the Outlaw Half in 2015, he actually told me I was stupid. After I had decided not to train with his group any more, I reckon he thought I was giving up. However, a few months later I went on to complete the Outlaw Half without his coaching, and, although I bumped into him regularly, he never made a comment about Outlaw.

His reply to my post, however, really got me riled. Seeing I'd hired James, this guy's comment was, 'Was my training too hard for you? You need an "I can" attitude, not an "I won't"!'

Well ... my blood boiled! How dare he imply that I didn't have the right attitude to my training! His training was never 'too hard', it was simply unrealistic and a totally old-fashioned, selfish approach. I cannot be 'selfish' and ignore what happens at home; I have parental duties that come top of my list and should be on anyone's list of priorities. Those who know me know I have the biggest 'I can' attitude of anyone! If ulcerative colitis wasn't going to beat me, if having an ileostomy wasn't going to stop me, then one man's bad attitude wasn't going to beat me either. Negative people have no place in your life – all they do is drag you down by telling you what you cannot do. Well, I *can* be an Ironman. Just watch!

Needless to say, I did send him a personal note of thanks for his help and assistance with my swimming at the outset, but I never got a reply. I think that shows the true colours of a person. He doesn't exactly shun me at the pool, but he never bothers to say hello any more unless I make the first move – it's as though I don't exist. Well, I think that's a shame. Now I am focussing on positivity and having the right people around me, who believe in me 100 per cent.

One aspect of having the right people around you is recognising how training with others can boost your training. I've buddied up with Al for some months now, and I can honestly say that having someone to run, bike

TEN

and swim with has definitely had a positive impact on my training. In the pool we compare our paces, we take turns at leading out (although I usually lead and he drafts along behind me), but it's being out on the road that gives the biggest rewards. Al is a great hill climber on the bike – he just powers up non-stop, whereas I get to a point, then have to stop and push the bike up the really steep hills. He will wait at the top and tease me about making it up the hill – it makes training fun. That's what makes the difference; if you're having fun, you put in the effort without seeing it as a tough slog.

Al and I have different running styles too, but this is helping both of us. My strategy is run/walk – I run for a distance, sometimes with a little push on speed to a set point like a tree or a lamppost, then walk to a set point. This gives my body time to recover, whether it's my legs or my lungs that need it. However, Al's style is to just keep going – as he says to me, 'Only stop for coffee.' I was wondering if I was holding him back with my run/walk strategy, but it was nice to hear him tell me that running with me makes him quicker. Well, running with him makes me run longer! So it's win/win!

Looking at our Strava statistics over time (Strava is an online program that takes the data from your GPS watch and tracks your pace etc), even as we don't always get to run together, it's interesting to see Al's approach means he is quicker than me on 5km and 10km distances, but when you look at the longer distances, my times are better. I use Strava all the time to record my activities; it's a great way to see my progress and also to compare myself with others. Plus your friends can watch and comment on your progress, which is all extra motivation and encouragement.

Probably the biggest downside of having a training partner of the opposite sex is the effect it has on others, which can be counter-productive to the training. Your training partner becomes your best friend, you share a common goal and are so pleased to see their development. We chat all the time about targets, runs, ride routes etc. It's like they are part of your family. But from the outside, people can feel excluded and become a little envious of the time you spend together. Craig got really upset that I spent so long chatting with Al about triathlons; I suppose I never saw it from his perspective and understand how it might look if the roles were reversed. I know Al has had the same issues.

Sadly, this has meant Al and I cannot run together unless we are in a group with others. It seems a bit extreme, but it's important that the feelings of those at home are considered. This is really hard, because a training partnership doesn't have a group dynamic, and trying to arrange for others to come out and run with us at 6.30am every week is pretty much impossible. So we end up resorting to running solo. We both go out and train at the same time, but in different locations; we live in different towns, so we each run where we live. I've lost my training buddy, and with it my mojo and my confidence to run early in the morning.

A woman going out running alone in the dark at 6.30am in the winter just doesn't feel safe. This has had a bigger impact on my training. Trying to motivate myself to run is getting harder and harder with the cold, dark mornings. I am leaving it later to go out, but then worry about time pressure to get my run done and get showered before work. This isn't good, and I wish I had my training partner back. Especially as he has now told me that he and

TEN

his wife are going to be moving abroad for three years from the end of February, and we've decided to run a half-marathon together before he goes.

I was mentally preparing to lose my training buddy in February, but now I feel that I've lost him in December, before I was ready to go solo.

So it is timely that I hired James as my coach. With him on board, my training is coming on amazingly. Having someone to set the training plan for me to follow makes it so much easier for me to fit in. In a typical week, I swim on Monday and have a short run; Tuesday is strength and conditioning; Wednesday is my long run day, and this is ramping up week by week with the Portland Coastal Half Marathon coming up on 7 February as my first race of the season. Thursday is bike day – on the turbo at the moment, as the weather has been so awful. Friday means another swim and a one-hour 'recovery' run. To me, no run is about recovery – it's all just hard work! Then it's a long bike ride on Saturday morning and rest day on Sunday. I have found that my best time to train is very early morning. On Monday, Wednesday and Friday I am out to start my swim or run at 6.30am – so that means it's a 5am start. Other days I am up early and train before anyone else in the house wakes up.

As for the bike turbo sessions, I am using the time to catch up on TV programmes I've missed, usually of one-hour duration – it makes the training go by much quicker. It's all about training the muscles, so if I can keep the mind occupied, then that's much easier. I cannot wait until the weather dries up and I can take my new bike out on the road. I've challenged Al to do the bike and run brick session at Lynmouth, which I did in the Tri the Beast triathlon. A brick session is when you do two disciplines back to back, usually the bike session followed immediately by a run.

The Tri the Beast bike route is a tough 30 miles of hills on the bike and a 10km lumpy run. We just have to try to get this in before Al leaves the country.

Chapter Eleven

CHRISTMAS IS now over, and I actually had four days' rest period. Yes, rest is as important as the training. I've been struggling with pain in my ankle in recent weeks, and this short break has given it time to rest up. I've no idea what's causing the pain: it could have been my new running shoes, but I will have to test this theory. For now, I have reverted to my old shoes. My long runs are now up to 13.6km, and this took me 1 hour 31 minutes. I run along the estuary to Crow Point in Braunton. The further I run, the more new places I am finding. Based on this run time, I should be able to run a marathon (42km) in something like five hours, but that's not allowing for me to slow down as I tire. Let's see what the results of the half-marathon on 7 February bring. My target time for this event is 2 hours 30 minutes.

It's funny how your mindset towards training changes the more you get involved. I now have a training programme that often requires two disciplines a day. This week my training started with a swim and run, knowing I'd never get a run in during the day due to work commitments. I decided to do the run straight after my swim, before work ... when did this lazy couch potato of a woman become so focussed to do this before work?

Whilst it felt good to get two sessions out of the way, so I could get on with the day, James has subsequently told me I really ought to have two meals between the sessions so that my body is recovered and refuelled. I am learning all the time; it's not just about the quantity of training you have to do, but the way you structure it to get the best results from your body.

* * * * *

James is increasing my mileage week on week now, as I have the London Marathon on 24 April as my first A race. I have two short runs of 30–45 minutes per week and one long run. This week I've got nine miles (14.5km) to run. Fortunately, I have some great friends in the tri club who are happy to run with me, so I've arranged to meet Donna Marriott on Saturday at 7.30am. We start early so we can incorporate Park Run at Rock Park in Barnstaple into our run.

At 7.30am I arrive at the park to find not only Donna, but Joyce Mulholland and Caroline Jones, plus Ginny the dog: what a great running team! Ginny is attached to Donna by a running belt and she's raring to go; it's funny to watch the dog dragging as hard as she can to run whilst Donna is trying to keep her back to a steady warm-up pace. Ginny is clearly more excited about regular running than I am.

We head out down the Tarka Trail at a steady Zone 1 to Zone 2 pace. Zone 1 is like a gentle jog, and Zone 2 is just picking up the pace a bit – there's no way I will be running flat out at Zone 5! It's good to run with the girls; being able to chat whilst we run helps me to forget

ELEVEN

about my legs and run further without having to walk. I do still walk a couple of times, especially when I need to take on some nutrition. I've run three miles down the Tarka Trail before turning and heading back. We get back to Rock Park with a few minutes to spare before the 5km Park Run begins; this will be the last three miles of our planned nine-mile run.

For the first time ever, with Caroline running beside me, I manage to run the whole 5km without walking, probably because I was well and truly warmed up before we started. I cannot wait to see my Strava statistics from this run, and even more so my Park Run result.

Later in the day, the results are in. I was just one second off my Park Run personal best time, and that was after running nine miles. This training is doing good, and having friends to run with makes a huge difference.

Next week I've got my first local event of the season: Braunton 10.

* * * * *

Feeling very excited today. This is my first event of the season, and not only do I have my training buddy here to run with me, but also a number of my tri club mates. The start is at the Braunton Athletics Centre, and we're all lining up under the inflatable start line. We hang back towards the back of the pack, because there's nothing more demoralising than watching everyone run past you. A little group of us run at a nice steady pace, whilst the faster road runners shoot off into the distance. To me, this is just another training run; it's about getting into a rhythm and concentrating on my cadence.

James is now asking me to weigh myself before and after a run, so we can calculate what my body is burning on a long run. He's particularly keen to make sure we calculate my nutrition requirements.

Braunton 10 is described as being an 'undulating' course. My idea of undulating and that of the organisers is clearly very different – this has two really big hills. By the end of the run, I've lost 5lbs in weight! Between now and Ironman in July, James reckons I will lose another stone, and that's just the 'extra' benefit of training. If he's right, I should be quicker on the bike, just by being lighter.

* * * * *

I cannot believe how quickly time has flown. I'm now in Portland, a small island at the end of a causeway from Weymouth, and I'm about to take part in my first really long event of the year: the Portland Coastal Half Marathon. I cannot believe I'm running a half-marathon. Me?! The girl who hated cross-country running at school and would do absolutely anything to get out of it. The girl who used to need an inhaler for asthma attacks. Here I am, about to run a half-marathon! I keep repeating this to myself, but that, I think, is to convince myself that it's really me doing this.

As we drive to Portland from north Devon, we encounter the most terrible flooding as Storm Imogen is on its way in. Saturday's weather forecast was awful, but today, Sunday, it's meant to be clearer in the morning but closing in again in the afternoon. If that's not motivation to get this half-marathon done quickly, then I don't know what is.

It feels strange turning up at the registration hall completely unsupported by team-mates or family. Craig and the kids have gone off to Dorchester Dinosaur Museum, as the children find all the hanging around at

ELEVEN

events very boring. You can't blame them, really: they get to see me swim if it's a pool triathlon, then just about see me scoot off on the bike, and I'm gone for ages. The next time they would see me is at the finish line. So today, with a half-marathon ahead of me and a storm brewing, they definitely don't want to be hanging around. With Al's imminent move abroad, he's had to withdraw, as they are in the midst of packing up their house, so this final event that we were going to do together is now my solo event.

So I enter the hall and register. It seems more laid-back here than at a triathlon, I guess because you don't have to rack up your bike and set up all your transition kit. Here, where the start and finish are in the same place, I can just put my pack in a corner and leave it there until I finish.

Once I have pinned my race number on to my leggings and changed my mind several times as to whether or not to wear my long-sleeved running top over my trisuit, all that's left to do is put on my timing chip. Now, here's another novelty: I'm used to having the timing chip Velcroed around my left ankle for triathlon, but, as I'm only running this time, I have to attach the timing chip to my shoelaces. With my buff on my head as some small measure against the weather, I have never felt more togged up for an event than this.

This run has a very special feel to it for me, as a friend in the US, Christel Carr-Elliott, who also has an ileostomy, was recently involved in a hit-and-run incident. She'd spent the last year recovering from her stoma surgery and getting her life back together, and now she's been hit at speed and been left with broken hips in the road at night, and had to drag herself to the pavement to avoid being hit by other vehicles. Christel is an amazing marathon runner and an inspiration, and now someone has taken away her passion. It's humbling to think about how precious life is: all those with an ostomy that I have to come to know have been through tough times yet come out having their life back. Being able to run this half-marathon is something I am fortunate to be able to do – whether I am fast or slow. So I am dedicating this run to Christel. She will be my driving force for this event, no matter what the day brings.

The people running the full marathon distance line up first for their briefing, and they are off at 9am. I stand and watch, ready to race, and I've still got half an hour to kill. With no North Devon Tri Club team-mates here, I do feel more like this is a training run. Most of the time now I do my runs alone. This will probably help me around the event. Let's be honest, I am never going to win a race, so I am taking each event and enjoying it for what it is.

It's 9.30am and we're ready to start the half-marathon – 13.1 miles. To date, this is my longest run since getting seriously into my training. As usual, I hang back; the last thing I want is to feel like I am being pushed to run faster than I need to at the front. We run around the Sailing Academy and very soon turn off up a muddy trail. This is how it's going to be today – muddy! We climb for two miles up a slippery trail path, and we're all walking. It's steep, but I'm confident that this is the worst of it. How wrong I am soon proven to be.

As we spread out, there are strings of people ahead of me, like a snake writhing along the narrow path, and there are still a handful behind me. It's trail running all the way, and some parts of the Portland Coastal Path remind me of my training ground out at Braunton and Crow Point. I get to an arrow to turn right, but hesitate as there are a number of possible directions. Three other

ELEVEN

runners join me and we follow our instincts. Only when we meet a residential road do we realise it was the wrong direction, so we retrace our steps and eventually find the right course around the prison. Feed station one appears, and we've already covered nearly three miles – that was quick, I thought.

We head down a steep trail with stunning views. All that climbing was worth it for these views over the coast of Weymouth. From the bottom of the trail, I join two ladies and we run together amiably. This trail turns to rock climbing as the route takes us through a terrain of boulders. Thankfully the yellow arrows sprayed on to the rocks keep us on track. As we head towards the lighthouse in the distance, we run across very high and exposed ground.

Now the weather is really starting to hammer us. With the storm coming in across the sea, the headwinds of 70–80mph make it difficult to run. With the rain lashing down as I try to traverse the clifftop, I'm being blown uphill, sideways. The effort needed just to stay in a straight line takes more out of my legs. The sea is being whipped up to a monstrous fury below us, and the sea foam is blowing across us right up here at Portland Bill. Never have I been in the midst of such natural power out on a run.

Crabbing sideways across the exposed top, I make it to the second feed station, where I manage to munch down a handful of salted crisps. The last thing I want is cramp, and, with my compromised digestion, I have to be on top of my electrolytes. At every feed station, I refuel my water bottle with a hydro tab. This is crucial for me.

Running uphill again across exposed ground, we have so much rainwater up here that we are running on slippery, boggy ground. As our feet slurp through the mud, we are whipped by the wind and sea foam. The wind from this point onwards is relentless – no let-up whatsoever. It's great, then, to see the third feed station, and how I missed out on the chocolate here I just do not know. Actually, I do know: I wasn't here quick enough.

It's now all downhill and flat; running through more rocky terrain, but this time on a path, I come to the top of steep steps carved into the hillside. It's a long way down, and I feel for the full-distance marathon runners who are now coming back the other way. Everything I have just been through, so have they, and now they have to go back and do it all again in reverse in this weather. They already look exhausted. I'm glad I'm not going back the other way.

At the bottom of the hill, it's now all flat along Chesil Beach for 3km – that sounds easy in my head after what I've just run, but, with the strong winds, even this last stretch is tough. I'm feeling completely exhausted, and my body just wants to stop moving. I've never found it so hard to run. A few dog-walkers who have braved the weather call out, 'Well done, nearly there!' It feels like I am running through treacle. I resort to a very slow final stint of run/walk strategy until I cross the finish line with a last burst of energy. I was determined to run the last bit no matter what, and it was great to see the friendly face of a fellow ostomate, Anne Marks, who I'd met through the Ostomy Lifestyle Athletes group, and had come out to see me finish.

Strava records my moving time as 3 hours 2 minutes, although I know I've been out there for three and a half hours. The weather was tough, but I don't think I took on enough nutrition, which is why I was wilting at the

ELEVEN

end. That's something to try more on my next long run – which will be on Friday.

I finish the day feeling great – exhausted, but still feeling great. Not only do my legs feel good, with no aches or pains, but it's a great medal to start 2016 for me.

* * * * *

Everything has gone barmy in the last couple of days, all in a positive way. A couple of weeks ago I spent the day filming with the BBC. I so want to help inspire others that I had made contact with Andrea Ormsby at BBC South West with a view to getting some interest, maybe, in a documentary about my endeavours to become an Ironman. The BBC are interested in doing a news piece on me for the TV on the regional programme *BBC Spotlight* as well as for BBC Radio Devon. I brought my coach, James Lapish, in on this, as I knew it would add an extra dimension to the story for Andrea. For a day, we had fun filming at Saunton. We started with an interview on the patio of the Saunton Sands Hotel, with the beach as a backdrop. I am eternally grateful to Kelly and Peter Brend for allowing us the use of their hotel as a venue.

We spent the morning down on the windy beach, where James and I took a training session to a fun level, running at the camera as Andrea lay on the damp sand, leaping over her at the last moment. She would definitely get some great action shots from that angle. Close-up shots and long-distance shots, James and I just ran back and forth along the beach – not quite a proper training session, but a giggle anyway.

A kit change, and we put on our cycling gear. We used Croyde as our location, as it was nice and close to the hotel and the roads were not too busy. Initially James gave me some instruction about how to get the most efficient line and speed through a corner; clearly it was the little things that were going to make my cycling smoother. We took it gently down the twisting descent from the hotel down into Croyde. This was going to be quite a day, as it was the first time I'd taken my new bike out.

As Andrea set up her camera on a bend, to enable her to film us going in either direction, James led me up the hill that we had just come down. I am no mountain goat, and I hate riding up hills with a passion. I just didn't seem to have enough power in my legs to make the wheels turn at a decent pace to get up the hills, and I am prone to getting off and walking. With the camera rolling, I was going to have to dig deep and try to get up this hill. As we built up speed on the flat run-up to the hill, the bike felt so light; at the incline, the wheels were still turning and they kept turning. I could not believe how light and easy this bike was to ride.

Before I knew it I was at the top of the hill, and I hadn't struggled at all. Amazed at this, I was coming to realise how important having the right equipment is to performing well. I know anyone can compete in a triathlon, but having the above-average bike really had made this feel so different. After a spot of lunch, we headed to the hotel's indoor pool to do some swim filming. I am very lucky to have had James with me all day, as whilst we were only doing short clips, for the camera, he was actually coaching me on technique in all three disciplines, all day. He also had to do a one-to-one interview to camera, and I stepped away whilst he did it. When I heard what an honest and heartfelt interview he had done, I blushed at his kind words. I'm glad he feels so positively about coaching me.

ELEVEN

Knowing that we'd wrapped up the filming, it was then a waiting game until it was aired on TV, and I was told that BBC Radio Devon wanted to do a piece on my story and wanted to do a live radio interview with me. On Thursday 11 February, I was sat in my car listening in to BBC Radio Devon at 7.25am, waiting for the producer to patch me through to the studio.

It was surreal sitting in the car hearing Simon Bates introduce the piece about my journey: Simon Bates – the Radio 1 DJ who I used to listen to all the time when I was growing up. Just hearing his voice conjures up memories of 'Our Tune' on Radio 1, and now here he was talking about me.

At lunchtime on *BBC Spotlight*, a shortened version of the film footage was due to go out after the national news. Without a TV at the office, I headed to the TV shop on Barnstaple High Street, who kindly put the right channel on for me to watch. Of course, this got them intrigued and I ended up watching the news item with the salesman and a shopper – how embarrassing.

The longer video version was due to go out on the 6.30pm news, but I was attending a women's night at the Bike Shed in Barnstaple at that time, so I'd have to watch it when I got home later. As I watched the time tick by, I knew it was going out on air. I sat at the front of the presentations and tried to concentrate on the speaker, who was explaining to us about power output. My mobile phone, which I had on silent in my pocket, suddenly came alive; it kept buzzing and vibrating every time a text message or notification popped up on my screen. I hadn't told many people that this was about to go on air, so they had probably spluttered over their dinner when they saw me on the screen.

During the break in the presentations, I checked my phone and found one lady had reached out to me via Twitter, wanting to interview me for her blog on Triathlove. I had to step out and let her know I could chat the following day. This was all getting so exciting, and I loved that it wasn't just the ostomy industry that wanted to hear what I was doing, but the triathlon world did too. On the same day, a lady who organises a stoma group meeting in Crediton also emailed me, as someone had seen the news item and told her about it. I was now signed up as their guest speaker in August. A surge of warmth ran through me as I realised that by sharing my story, I was helping other ostomates to realise that they can do so many positive things with a bag.

Chapter Twelve

JAMES HAS me down for a 19km run today; so, as Craig and the kids have to go into Barnstaple, the plan is for me to run from there back home to Ilfracombe via the quieter country roads, which are, unfortunately, also the hillier roads. Running this distance, I'm not going to be able to carry sufficient fluids on me, so we hide one of my water bottles in a hedge six miles into my route, making a mental note of the visual markers around it so I can find it on the way back. I am then dropped off in Barnstaple as the kids laugh at the prospect of me running all that way whilst they're off shopping.

I leave the Tesco car park and head out of town at an easy pace, crossing the new bridge over the estuary, and head out through a residential route through Pilton. I don't run with headphones or music, as I cannot race with headphones, so part of the training with long runs is to get accustomed to the solitude. As I run down the street, cars are passing me, but then one car stops slap bang in the middle of the road, with a queue of vehicles behind it. The woman driver winds down her window as if she's about to ask for directions.

'I just have to say I think what you're doing is really impressive. Well done, and keep on going.'

I'm totally flabbergasted, but I thank her with a beaming smile; this lady has just made my day. My story is reaching people and already having an impact. My motivation to keep on running is sky-high. I carry on with a spring in my step.

The journey home is extremely tough, with lots of big hills to climb. I do have to walk some of them, and it's good to see the halfway point in the distance by the visual markers. As I reach the six-mile point, I find my drink bottle is still tucked away safely inside the hedgerow. I know that the last three miles into Ilfracombe will all be downhill, as I've cycled this route many times. So, pushing up these last few hilly miles, I know it's almost near the end. I've also been testing out some home-made energy bars.

Because of my reduced absorption of calories and fluids, I need to be very aware of my nutrition. Many of the energy bars in shops or online I find either have the taste and texture of cardboard, or have ingredients like nuts, meaning that, whilst great fuel, my body simply cannot digest them. Nuts and fruit skins are potentially liable to cause a blockage in my ileostomy. The consequences of this I have experienced before. A blockage can be excruciatingly painful, leaving me doubled up in pain. All I can do is drink fluid and hope the blockage passes quickly. If not, I might have to be taken to hospital. So, rather than take the risk with traditional energy bars, I have taken natural ingredients and ground them down into a form that is easily digestible. Using ingredients such as fresh fruit and raw cacao, these cold pressed bars pack a great calorific content, and I've added a natural ingredient

TWELVE

that settles the stomach. So today's run was my first test of the bars.

* * * * *

An early start, and I am buzzing from an early-morning swim at the pool. An endurance programme of 2.2km took me 1 hour 9 minutes, which for me isn't too bad really. After lunch, it's time to put in what James calls a 'recovery run'. Well, this isn't a recovery run, but a run I'll need to recover from. I only have to run for 45 minutes, but after just 10 minutes, as I start to pick up the pace, I start to feel a pain in my left calf. I continue running, thinking I can run this feeling off, but before long I pull up to rub the painful leg, realising that perhaps this isn't one that I can just run through. In the end, I do manage to run for 40 minutes, but it's very much a run with walking sections. In fact, it hurts more to walk than to run. Not only does my leg hurt, but I am also getting sore around my stoma.

I don't usually have to consider my stoma, as for me it is now so normal that I tend to forget it's there. However, today I've been wearing a different type of stoma bag. I have opted for a one-piece system, as the material it is made from was ideal for my swim; but, by this afternoon, with running trousers and a bumbag clipped around it, I can feel the intense pain and soreness that comes from output getting on to my skin under the base flange.

Thankfully, this is only a short run of just under 6km, and I manage to hobble back to the office, where I am glad to change and put on a new stoma bag. For those with an ostomy, output getting on to your skin is not at all pleasant – the acidic nature of the output (as it hasn't been through a large intestine) burns your skin. If it stays on the skin for any length of time, it can eat away the skin and leave it sore and bleeding. Running and competing with a stoma, the problem isn't just that it's there and something to consider: there are so many more issues an ostomate has to deal with. Finding the right stoma bag system that works for you and your lifestyle is a big part of that. I've learned that a one-piece system – i.e. the whole bag and flange is one complete unit – works well for me under a swimming costume, but doesn't work for running.

The material that is used for the bags, from various manufacturers, could be more water-resistant or could be soft. However, the base of them is made from hydrocolloid, which is designed to absorb fluid. That's fine for everyday wear, but for swimming it just goes gummy around the edges. So I set out to find a solution to my swimming needs. That's when I come across the silicone flange extenders from Trio Ostomy Care, which are like a second skin – so soft and fine that when I put them over my base plate/flange, it stops any water getting under it and solves the issue of going all gummy.

After a disappointing run, I make a call to the organisers of the Virgin London Marathon. I've been focussing my training on increasing the run distances for my place in this marathon in April, but I've been getting a little concerned. The lady who told me she was transferring her place in the marathon to me has gone rather quiet, and I've not heard anything for some time. She told me she had sent all the necessary paperwork to VLM to get the place transferred and that I should be hearing from them. Now, after several weeks, she has vanished. We'd known each other through some closed Facebook groups for ostomates, but now she appears to have closed her account and I've no other way of contacting her.

TWELVE

I call the helpdesk with her details and mine and explain the situation. I am therefore devastated when the man on the end of the phone tells me that the place is still listed in her name, and in actual fact she isn't allowed to transfer her place to me to run on her behalf. She would have been told that at the time of her applying, and again when she approached them to transfer it to me.

I hold back the tears as I thank the man for his help. Hanging up, I crumble. I am totally gutted. I've been training heavily for the London Marathon, and now it's all for nothing! How can someone who knew how important this was to me just lie and disappear? Did she know she couldn't transfer the place? Did she close her Facebook account to save herself the embarrassment of telling me she'd got it wrong? As someone who had supposedly run the London Marathon twice before, she would have known how hard the training would be for this, and yet she stopped replying to my messages and then closed her account so that she couldn't be contacted.

I feel hollow and let down. My first big A race of the season now doesn't exist. Had I known I wouldn't have a place in the London Marathon, I would have been training differently, focussing on Ironman. James had had concerns about me doing both the London Marathon and Ironman in the first place, and had designed my training plan to fit my race schedule. Now we would have to change the plans and try to recover the lost time, focussing on my swimming and cycling.

I suppose I should look on the positive side: I've already bagged the Portland Coastal Half Marathon this year as part of my training and am much further ahead with my running than I would have been had I not had the London Marathon on my calendar. Whilst I could still get a place in the Manchester Marathon, which would be two weeks before the London Marathon date, I've decided not to compromise my training for Ironman. I had wanted to know in my own mind that I could complete a marathon before I got to Ironman UK in Bolton, but I am going to have to put that thinking out of my head now and just hope I can train well enough for Ironman Staffordshire 70.3 and Bolton and believe I can do it. Ironman UK is my big A race of the year, and that is clearly in my sights.

*****

With the rollercoaster of recent events with my injured calf and the lost place in the London Marathon, I've been feeling very emotional. I am sure part of this is the lack of being able to train due to my injury; it's still hurting when I walk, and I'm not recovering as quickly as I thought I would. This is potentially going to stop me running in this weekend's Castle Hill Corker, a fun ten-mile trail run that a number of my tri club mates are doing. It will be the first event we've done together this year, and, after the disappointment of the London Marathon, I really need a boost. I trust the judgement of my coach implicitly and must remember what I am ultimately training for. I want to be an Ironman.

However, I know that a big part of my emotions today is because in five days' time my training buddy, Al, is flying off to live abroad for three years. Whilst I knew this day was coming, it's been made so much harder by the fact that we've not been able to train together, and we weren't able to run the Portland Coastal Half Marathon together as we had planned. He has become my buddy, a great friend, and I've not had the opportunity to say goodbye to him before he goes. I was once told that your

TWELVE

training partner becomes like a brother or sister to you. I've found this is true, the bond you have. We've spent many hours cycling, running and swimming together, with a shared goal of improving to compete in triathlons. We understand what drives each other, and we rejoice in each other's successes.

I suppose spouses of triathletes who have training partners must all feel some sense of being 'left out', but there has to be trust and a recognition of the commitment this individual is putting into their training. I know from first-hand experience that having a training partner makes a huge difference to your drive and commitment to training. They encourage you, and they push you in a way that your friends and family cannot because they've not lived through the pain of training; and they celebrate with you, no matter how big or small the achievement. When we put in so much time and effort into our training, an occasional 'Well done' is all we need to hear.

* * * * *

Despite the recovering leg, I manage to get in a turbo session on my bike. Thankfully, I had popped in to Bike It over the weekend to get my saddle changed. The one that came on my Giant Envie is just so uncomfortable – it's as slim as a razor blade and so hard. I'd never be able to concentrate on cycling. I've taken my old comfortable saddle off my Peugeot Audax and switched it on to my new bike. Now it feels like I'm sitting in an old comfy chair, and my backside is grateful.

The turbo session is a test to see how my damaged calf bears up. As it turns out, by having my feet clipped on to the bike, it's my quads and glutes that are doing all the work, not so much my calf muscles. I manage, therefore, to do 90 minutes, including 20 minutes down on the aero bars.

In the morning, I was also in the pool at 7am for a 2.6km endurance swim. I definitely enjoy the endurance sets. I'm getting to know some familiar faces in the lanes now too. It's a nice way to meet people. Most are really considerate, and if I catch up with them in the lane, they will wait at the top and let me pass them. There's only one man who gets into the lane for about 15–20 minutes and seems to think he owns it. He's even swum over my arms when I've pushed off the wall at the end. He's extremely rude and 'huffs and puffs' about others in the lane. He's in for such a short amount of time, he's a real hindrance to my concentration. It's probably wrong of me to give in to a bully, but he's not worth the frustration, so I swim in the next lane when he turns up.

My calf muscle still hasn't got much better, so I've had to find a physio. James wants me to get it seen, because, as it's not healing, this will hold back my training; we've lost enough swim and bike time already and cannot afford to have me out of action. After asking friends for recommendations, I make an appointment to see Andrew Buller. Andrew is a very professional and attentive young physio/sports masseur in Barnstaple. He asks me if I can roll up my trouser leg so he can see the injured calf; to my horror I realise that I am so inappropriately dressed for this, wearing my tight-fitting leather trousers. With a bit of pushing and pulling, I get the trouser leg up to my knee. From doing some basic exercises for him, he quickly establishes that I have a grade 1 to grade 2 strain, where the ligament meets the gastrocnemius muscle. This sounds bad enough, but I count myself lucky when he tells me that a grade 3 would have been a rupture, so that

TWELVE

would have really put my training and possibly my races out of reach.

The treatment starts straight away with some intense massage. My own definition of massage is something slightly pressured and relatively enjoyable, but this is something altogether different. I've never had a sports massage, and it's worlds away from being 'enjoyable'. Pressing deep into the muscle, the massage feels more painful than the injury is. Andrew explains how this deep pressing will break down the fibres and get blood back into that area to heal. I can already envisage the bruises that I will have tomorrow in this area, but at least this will speed up the recovery rather than just leaving it to heal slowly on its own. I'll just have to wait and see if I can walk tomorrow.

* * * * *

It's been a month since my calf injury, and so much has happened in this short time. Perhaps it is fate that meant I wasn't going to be running in the London Marathon, considering my calf strain. In the last two weeks I've only been out running twice: the first time was a gentle three-minute jog/two-minute walk, to get the leg working and check it's not going to go 'ping' again. At the end of the 30-minute run/walk, I head back to the hotel where I am staying and I feel that awful pull in my calf muscle again. Oh no – has it gone again? Thankfully, a day later it's feeling better; perhaps it was just rebelling at being put to work again after three weeks of only running in water with no impact.

James suggested that I do water running whilst my leg was healing, and my physio had agreed it was a good, low-impact approach. It meant the rest of my 'running muscles' and hip flexors would still be exercised. I must admit I did feel a bit of a wimp in the swimming pool doing this. Whilst I couldn't swim in the lanes as usual, I had to run backwards and forwards across the deep end of the general swimming pool. In amongst the swimmers who use the pool for just keeping fit, I looked like someone who didn't even know how to swim. I reminded myself that this technique had been used by many professionals before they raced.

A few weeks later, I am back out on the roads again, as the leg is strengthening and it's great to get out and complete a 45-minute run around Ilfracombe, which is not exactly flat, and the leg is feeling fine, thank goodness. With this injury and work trips getting in the way, I feel like my training programme has been derailed a bit. I was religiously doing all my training sessions, eight times a week – but, being away on two consecutive weekends, my training has become more sporadic. I'm trying my best to keep on top of the sessions. Whilst staying up in Birmingham, I was committed to getting back on track with my training, so I took my bike and turbo trainer with me and set it up in my hotel room. The weather was surprisingly sunny, but I hadn't packed my crash helmet so couldn't take advantage of the area I was staying in. However, the hotel did have a leisure centre attached to it, so I used the pool instead for an hour of water running.

Having returned from Birmingham, I'm back on the road again, heading to Manchester for the Bike Expo/Tri Expo. I spend three days there on an exhibition stand with a couple of friends, promoting their business. The stand is swamped, and, particularly on the second day of the show, we find ourselves talking non-stop. By the end of

TWELVE

the day, we are almost hoarse from shouting over the top of the David Lloyd spin class that has been pumping out beside us, and we are all missing our training. Richard is a cyclist and Simon is a personal trainer and Ironman, so what do three athletes do after a long day on their feet? We head to the David Lloyd Leisure Centre next to our hotel for some therapeutic training, of course. Richard and I hit the bikes, and Simon heads off to the treadmill. I really am feeling like a true athlete now, with experienced people like these alongside me. I'm not the mum who is, in their words, a gym bunny. I really am seen as an equal. Dedication to training does put you into a different realm of exercise; it's not exercise, it's training.

At the end of day three, we all head home with rough voices and big grins on our faces. The weekend has been a great success, and I've met with the organisers of the Snowdonia Slateman triathlon that I am competing in later in May. Damian, the cameraman who filmed me earlier in the year for my sponsor, is also here and we manage to show the organisers the showreel of what we've done to date on my story, and they are hooked. They give Damian permission to have his own film crew out on the Snowdonia Slateman course to continue documenting my progress. Usually this privilege is only granted to Channel 4 and Eurosport in the restricted zones such as the transition area, but the organisers have even offered to take one of the crew out with them on their boat on to the lake when I swim.

* * * * *

The Snowdonia Slateman Savage is going to be a killer – I just know it. Last year I came up to Snowdonia with a bunch of tri club friends and I took on the Snowdonia

Slateman, just the sprint triathlon; that was enough. But here I am again, stupidly, back in the hotel in Snowdonia preparing to take on the Savage. This is two days of racing: on Saturday I've got the sprint distance race, then on Sunday it's going to be the Olympic distance one. Wishing to constantly push myself, and having watched my friends do the double last year, I want to give this a try and I have, yet again, been swept along by the enthusiasm of my friends who are racing again too.

As I open the curtains on Saturday morning, the heavy grey clouds are not what I wanted to see. Yesterday, I spent the day riding little stretches of the Llanberis Pass for Damian and the film crew from Into Productions for another video for Trio Ostomy Care. They are going to be following me for the whole weekend. The day had been bright and promising, and having my pal Samera Ismael with me made it even more enjoyable. We'd had to drive up to the top of the quarry to film up there too. This is part of the Olympic course, and Samera had raced it before. The scenery is stunning from the top of the quarry, harsh grey slate contrasting with the lush green woodland surrounding it.

After an early, hearty breakfast, I wheel Piston out of the hotel with a load of other competitors who are also staying there. Great big raindrops begin to fall as I walk the short distance to the side of Lake Padarn, where we are going to swim. Everyone has concerns about the water temperature, as it's notoriously cold. There's no time today to think about this: I have to get racked up. There's no space for bags to be left by the bike at this event, so everything we need has to be laid out by the bike and bags dropped in a safe area. This means everything is going to be soaked before we have even started.

TWELVE

I join the crowd of wetsuited competitors who are grouping up by the lake, ready to be called in for their wave. The older age groups usually go in last, but here I seem to be going in before some of the younger ones. We are called forward into the water. It's freezing! I'm not wearing any neoprene footwear or gloves, but I have put on a neoprene hood under my swim cap to help prevent 'brain freeze'. We have only a minute to wade out into deeper water to the floating start line, but I cannot get my breath. Letting water down into my wetsuit, this usually gives me time to warm up a layer of water inside it – but from the moment I get down and let the water in, we are already being counted down for the start.

Swimming in such deep and cold water, the sheer terror overwhelms me. The horn blows and everyone is off. I cannot breathe, and I make a few strokes of breaststroke, hoping to get warm and start swimming properly. But it's not happening. I drop further and further back from the rest of the pack, with a kayak paddling beside me, which I put a hand up to grab. The kayaks are there to help anyone in trouble. I've hardly swum any distance and already I'm scared to death. My feet are going numb. I try again and still cannot put my face in the water; it's pitch black and ice cold. Why, oh why did I think I could do this?

The kayak stays near, and I continue around the first buoy. As I swim parallel to the shore, I can see the next wave of swimmers are already in the water, chasing me down. Now, not only am I panicking because of the cold and how slow I am, now I am at risk of being swum over by faster swimmers. I swim further out so they can pass me, adding more distance to my swim. After reaching the second buoy, I turn to shore as more and more people swim around me. There's only one exit point, so I'm inevitably going to get in someone's way.

As my hands reach out for the shallows of the bank, they touch the soft mud. I put my knees and feet down to stand up, only to find myself sinking in the sludge. Everyone is having the same problem as we grovel along in the soft, shifting silt until we reach the solid bank. Out of the water, we run to the transition and change on to the bike. The rain is pouring now, and it's a struggle to get my jersey and jacket on – they keep sticking to me. The route leads us up the Llanberis Pass at the base of Mt Snowdon. This is a straight-up-and-back route today, but it's a long, steady climb until we get over the top and descend to our turn point; then it's back up and over again. The descent is so beautiful, and, without having to push hard, I can take in the dramatic scenery, just hoping no sheep hop out in front of me.

The run is another stunning route, out across the far side of the lake and up through dense woodland. I love the trail run, but this is steep and I have to walk up some stretches. Once at the top, however, we are rewarded with spectacular views over the valley. The downward run is much more pleasurable, albeit technical as we dodge tree roots and hop from rock to rock. The final run across the field to the finish line is a wonderful feeling. Now all I have to do is repeat it all again tomorrow, but twice the distance.

Sunday's weather is an improvement. No longer is it pouring with rain, at least for the time being. Today Samera Ismael, Susan Standford and Lorrie Woolgar are racing the Olympic distance too, so it feels reassuring to have them with me as I rack up Piston. However, today I am more scared than I was yesterday. I feel sick, and, with

TWELVE

Aaron doing close-up shots of my face on camera, I'm doing my best to hold it together. The tannoy instructs all competitors to make their way across the field to the lake. I'm very subdued and cannot speak as I quietly follow behind Samera and Lorrie. Seeing me crying behind them, they immediately put their arms around me reassuringly.

After the panic attack in the water yesterday, I am seriously struggling to do this again today. The neoprene hood wrapped under my chin feels choking, and I feel like I cannot breathe. Never have I been so terrified. With the cameras still rolling, Samera and Lorrie get me doing star jumps to keep warm and refocus. The field is strewn with cowpats, and, as our bare feet accidentally step in them, Lorrie is kicking it all about like a mud bath. A fit of giggles comes over all of us as our wetsuits are splattered, but are about to get washed off shortly in the lake.

Stepping into the water, tears of panic fill my goggles. I am surrounded by a number of women who can see my distress, and I am touched by the support they give, offering to swim in slowly with me. I cannot hold anyone back from their race, and a big part of me wants to back out altogether. But I can't; I've come this far, and I have to face my fear and keep going.

Once we start, I take it slowly and roll gently side to side to make sure I have plenty of time to get my breath as I swim. By the time I reach the first buoy, which is now much farther out into the lake, I am calming down. Focus. Focus. Focus. I calm my breathing and slowly but surely get into a rhythm, but I still cannot put my face in the freezing cold water. As I exit the lake, the relief is overwhelming. I'm so pleased to have put that behind me. Now I can enjoy the rest of the race. Pumped up on adrenaline, I head up the Llanberis Pass again on Piston. Riders of all shapes and sizes come past me, but I am happy with my pace. As I reach the top of the Pass, I find I am now overtaking people who have had to get off and walk. Now is my time to fly. Piston feels as light as a feather as we descend down the winding road. At the bottom, today we make a left turn and head out along an undulating road. This is where the aero bars come into their own. My legs are powering along as I pass rider after rider shouting 'Coming through'. What a sensation.

The weather is a mixed bag. It's been a wet morning, and we get moments of sunshine and then sudden outbursts of rain and hail. Coming back to the transition area, my running shoes are wet through. Squelching into them, I make my way out on to the run course, which leads us along the road we've just ridden, but now cuts us up towards the slate quarries. I've not had any need to stop for a bag change this time, but as I climb up into the quarry I am bursting for the loo. There's no one behind me, but very little shrubbery to tuck behind. Ahead I spot a low gorse bush. I've no choice but to squat behind it. I thought my days of squatting behind bushes were long gone, but at least I now have an expert eye for opportune moments like this. I'm wearing a one-piece trisuit, so I've no option but to unzip the whole thing for a quick pee. As I zip up the suit again I hear a loud buzzing; looking around, I expect to find a swarm of bees in the sky. No bees! Just a drone! That was close; had the drone been a couple of minutes earlier, it would have caught me in all my glory!

Climbing to the top of the quarry is a relief, and, as the sun has now come out and beats down on my back, I take in the most stunning, lunar-like surroundings of

TWELVE

all the grey slate. This truly is the most beautiful event I have competed in. The downhill route joins the bottom of yesterday's course. As I cut across to the field running up to the finish, I see the iconic green and white trisuits of Samera and Lorrie, who have already finished. They've come out on to the final part of the run to join me for the last stretch. Three North Devon Tri ladies running side by side is the epitome of the bond I've come to cherish.

    I cross the finish line. I am a Savage!

Chapter Thirteen

IN PREPARATION for Ironman UK at Bolton, I have booked myself into doing Ironman Staffordshire 70.3. This being an Ironman event with two different transition locations, I'd heard all kinds of stories about the bus service to get athletes to the right place at the right time. So I am confronting this event with some trepidation. I have no tri club colleagues or any family and friends coming up to support me at this event, so I really am going solo. I am in two minds as to whether this is a good or a bad thing. On the negative side, I am facing a whole new experience without anyone around me to reassure me, or to ask their opinion or advice. I am going to have to work this all out for myself and trust my instinct, and a Half Ironman race is not something you can afford to get wrong. There's also the thought of the anti-climax when I cross the finish line and there won't be any family or friends to celebrate with me, no one I can hug and shout 'I did it' to.

I guess, therefore, I have to look at the positive side of having no support: this is a training day, albeit a very big training day. It's a day when I can become totally selfish and think only of what I need to do and when. I

THIRTEEN

can think about where I need to be and not have to worry about accommodating the needs of others who are not racing. I don't have the pressure of thinking the family will be bored when I'm out on the triathlon, and I can do whatever feels right without having to check it fits in with anyone else.

Sunday is race day, and I know it's going to be an early start, so I travel up to Stafford on Friday evening. I have no choice but to grab something to eat at a service station en route – so much for watching my nutrition! Arriving at the Premier Inn, I make a couple of trips up to my room. First I take my bike up; I manhandle it into the lift with the front wheel in the air, and squeeze it and myself out of a small lobby area on the second floor, only to find that my room key doesn't work and I have to make the awkward descent back down to reception. This really isn't the kind of start I had wanted for my biggest race to date.

I bring everything up to the room and start laying it all out on the floor. I know from the race pack that I will need to put all my cycle kit into a bag at Transition One (T1) and all my running kit into a bag at Transition Two (T2). However, these two transitions are about 20 miles apart. I write out a timetable of where I need to be and when on the Saturday, knowing that I need to park my car up and get a shuttle bus in the morning with my bike. I need to make sure I can be at the race briefing, which is in the Shugborough estate, and I also want to do the practice swim session at Chasewater. So I need to plan the day with military precision.

The following morning, the day before the race, I am up at 5am and make myself a quick porridge pot that I brought with me, knowing I'd be up and out long before the hotel breakfast would be served. The car journey to

Chasewater, where my bike, Piston, needs to be racked up, is 25 minutes' drive away. Pleased with my logistical planning, I arrive at the car park nice and early ready to catch the bus, which is a 15-minute journey to the actual Chasewater site where we will be swimming and racking up our bikes in T1. I am so early, I am one of the first in the car park and get a whole double-decker bus to myself. I'm pleased that it's all going to plan and it's not yet 7am. This is a really relaxed start to the day.

One other athlete gets on the bus, and we're driven to a drop-off point and told to walk down this little track. It looks like we've been dropped in the middle of nowhere. The other passenger and I chat amicably and follow the track until it comes into the back of the field where T1 is, and I get my first sight of the lake I will be swimming in tomorrow … it's huge! My nerves are kicking in already. We queue up behind a number of other early risers to get into transition, which is a fenced-off area where all the bikes will be left from now. As I near the front of the queue, I spot that the marshals are checking wristbands and numbers on the bikes. Oh, no! I am in the wrong place to register! I have to register at Shugborough, 20 miles away, where the finish line is, before I can enter this transition area! My heart races as I realise my mistake. I'd had this all timetabled out but had clearly misinterpreted something in the race pack. Because this is the start of the race, I'd made the mistake of thinking this was where we register too. I speak to the marshal at the entrance to T1, and he confirms that I have to get registered and collect my race numbers before I can drop my bike off.

I'm choking up; I'm alone. I've never done this before and now I'm panicking about the times I am meant to rack

THIRTEEN

up. The marshal tells me I can rack up any time before 4pm and the times given in the race pack were only a guide. Fuming at myself for making such a stupid mistake, I have to wheel my bike back past all the incoming competitors and back over the field, then down the lane to the drop point, and embarrassingly wait with my bike for the bus to come and get me. The transport manager recognises me from about 45 minutes earlier and looks quizzically at me. I explain my error and ask how far Shugborough is. That's when I learn that it's 20 miles away. So now I have to get back to my car, reload the bike on to the roof and drive another 25 minutes to the main venue, and start all over again.

Back at Shugborough, I park up in a field with hundreds of cars with bikes on their roofs; at least I'm in good company here. I head off to the triathlon village to find registration after what already feels like a long and frustrating morning. To heighten your excitement and urge to buy all things Ironman, the registration desks are at the end of a marquee that you find after meandering along the snake-like path amongst the expo stallholders. You can smell the testosterone and bravado amongst the stands, and hear the banter of exhibitors and even more excited chatter of the hundreds of competitors all heading for the same registration desks.

Finding my race number, I head to the appropriate check-in desk, just like at an airport, where I sign a disclaimer and I'm handed my Ironman rucksack filled with a variety of leaflets, together with my race numbers that are to be pinned on to my trisuit and race tattoos to be stuck on to my arm and leg, along with my three transition bags: red, blue and white. The lady at the check-in desk gives me an extra tattoo – an AWA gold standard one. My pack says I am an AWA gold standard too, but I've no idea what this means. I'm told it entitles me to special privileges for 'All World Athletes', who come in the top 1 per cent of their age category at Ironman events. I laugh at the error; I've never competed in an Ironman event before, let alone come in the top 1 per cent of anything.

Wandering back through the expo, I purchase the obligatory T-shirt and cap and head off to find some food before the race briefing at 12 noon. Starting to relax into the morning, I decide I might as well do everything I need to here before driving back to Chasewater to rack up in T1 again and stay for the practice swim in the lake.

The race briefing is packed solid, and you can feel the throb of humanity: every man and woman in the room is here with determination in their hearts to get round this course in the time limit. Everyone knows the race rules, but the chief referee reiterates them, and especially about the cut-off times within each discipline. This is going to be the most daunting, pressurised part of the race – making the cut-offs – but I am confident in my expected times and shouldn't need to worry about the cut-offs. I am hoping for a one-hour swim, four hours on the bike and two and a half hours for the run. Considering we have eight and a half hours to complete the whole event, I reckon I should finish in around eight hours with the transitions.

I'm starting to feel more confident now about everything – even, dare I say it, quite relaxed. The time pressure of this morning has gone now that I know I have the rest of the day to finish racking up.

Back at the car, I spread out all my transition bags on the grass and sort out what needs to go in each. It's more daunting doing this a day before the race, as anything missed out now won't be available to me tomorrow. Have

THIRTEEN

I got enough nutrition? What if it's a warm day? What if it's a wet day? I have to leave my bag here with everything for my run. I opt for stuffing 'options' into each bag: long-sleeve cycle jersey and short-sleeve cycle jersey, and more home-made energy bars than I am really likely to need. I leave a small bumbag in my run kit. That's one thing other triathletes don't have to think about: spare stoma bag supplies. Whilst I can manage my stoma output for a race to some degree with plant-based ingredients in my bars, there could be a time when it will all hit me and my stoma will go into overdrive. I don't want to get caught short on a half-marathon.

The transition tent is something new to me – usually I just have to rack up my bike on a bit of scaffolding and lay out my shoes, towel and race essentials on the ground. But here, my bag has to be hung on a peg just like a PE bag at primary school; I'm going to have to dash in one end of the tent, find my bag amongst all the other 2,000 and quickly change, stuff all my stripped/unwanted gear back in the bag and dash out at the other end of the tent. This is where having today to prepare and walk through the transition area settles my mind. As I hang my 'PE' bag on my numbered peg, I look around at the rows of racks. Never have I seen such a sight, and it strikes me what bedlam will ensue in here tomorrow.

The journey back to Chasewater feels familiar after this morning's fiasco. Chasewater is now getting busy; marshals check my wristband and race number on my bike before I am allowed access into the fenced transition area. There are hundreds of bikes already racked up. This event is monstrous! I cannot believe I am here and am one of the competitors. All those times watching Ironman on television, I've seen the vast rows of amazing racing bikes, and here I am on the inside of the fence, really a part of this now. The elites and pros have the lowest bib numbers, so when I look at the bikes racked up in numbers 1 to 20 I know that I am looking at some phenomenal bikes worth thousands of pounds, and the technology on them is amazing. No wonder these pros are fast. I think back to where I started on my old Peugeot Audax in my local race – this is worlds apart.

I rack Piston up on the bar and check the tyres; she's going to sit out here overnight in the rain, so there's no point leaving anything on the bike that's going to get sodden. It's dilemma time again: how much should I leave in my transition bag? Tomorrow we will have access to our bikes before the race, but not to our transition bags. Just like packing to go on holiday, I'm sure I've packed more into my transition bag than I really need. The art of a good transition is to get in and out as fast as possible. If I have only one set of clothes, in other words, make a decision today about what I will wear – that will save me from dithering on race day.

At 3pm I head to the waterside, as we're able to have a practice swim in the lake. Now, as I've said before, open-water swimming is my nemesis. I'm not afraid of what's in the water – it's the darkness of the water that freaks me out. I like the visibility of a swimming pool, but out here it's a whole different ball game.

Getting my wetsuit on, the nerves are kicking in and I can feel the tremble creeping up in my chest as I walk towards the water's edge. It's a gentle slope down the slipway into the water. There are plenty of people trying out the swim and canoes on the water to watch over us. Surprisingly, the water is warm. It's like bathwater. Well, more like the temperature of the swimming pool back

THIRTEEN

home. This means I am not breathless from the cold like I was at Snowdonia Slateman. Now I am only breathless from my nerves.

The water is a psychological battle for me. I'm not fast and find I need to breaststroke a little whilst I get my breathing under control. The canoes stay close, which is reassuring, and I remember my friend Kimberley's words: 'You can just bob.' I repeat this over and over in my head, and I start to relax and trust the buoyancy of my wetsuit and my ability to swim.

I only do a short practice, definitely not as far as the three buoys that most others are doing. I remind myself this isn't a race, and I'm in this enormous lake to get comfy and reassure myself that I can swim in this open water.

Dried and changed, I take the time to walk the transition route from swim to the bike. I visualise how the day will pan out tomorrow.

* * * * *

It's race day; it's early. Last night, I tried to get an early night after the ritual of putting my number tattoos on my arms. Being here on my own brings a mixed emotion of loneliness and focus. All I have to do today is follow my itinerary that I wrote out last night and visualise myself crossing that finish line. I know I can do this: I've prepared for it, and I know my times will all come in under the cut-offs.

I drive to Shugborough, where the finish line is. The finishers' chute red carpet leads through a corridor of barriers to the iconic Ironman gantry finish line. Later today I know I will come in under there. I may be alone, but I know many people are thinking of me today, none more so than my family and my coach, James Lapish.

I join the hundreds of other athletes who have arrived in this field of wet grass in the ridiculously early hours, all heading to the pick-up point for the shuttle bus that is to take us to Chasewater for the race start. All I have with me is my white plastic Ironman bag that will be stuffed with my daytime clothes before the start of the race, so they can be transported back to the finish line for me to pick up after I cross the line. For now, all it has in it are my wetsuit, my goggles, the Ironman swim cap that was in the registration pack, and my energy bars to put on the bike. I feel like I am travelling light and am nervous that I might have forgotten something, but it's too late now if I have.

The bus is filled with nervous triathletes; you can feel the tension. To break the silence, I chat to the man beside me, who is just as nervous as me, as it's his first Half Ironman distance too. The camaraderie of the triathletes relaxes me; I'm starting to believe I really am a triathlete. I'm here on this bus with loads of people who share the same dream of becoming an Ironman, and this Half Ironman distance is taking me one step closer.

The bus drops us by the path to the lake, somewhere I am now very familiar with after yesterday's chaotic planning. The nerves are now turning to excitement, and the chatter is getting louder. Whilst I am not due to be in the water until 8.25am, I still have to be finished in the transition area by 6am, as the elite triathletes will start their swim at 7am. This gives me a lot of 'hanging around' time, which is far too much thinking time for my liking. My head will be full of scenarios about the swim, which is the most daunting aspect for me.

After putting my energy bars and obligatory banana on the bike, it's time to watch the elite racing until the time comes for me to put my wetsuit on.

THIRTEEN

Half an hour before I am due to be in the water, I queue up for the toilets. Like at any festival, the queues for the Portaloos are very, very long, and then you have to remember to have some loo paper to hand because 2,000 nervous triathletes get through an awful lot of it. It seems my life still revolves around loo rolls even now.

This event has wave starts, whereby you enter the water at set times based on your age group and you self-seed yourself in that group based on your expected swim times. So the elites, professionals and younger age groups get in the water first. Then it's time for the older age groups in the later waves. I'm in the last wave as I'm 50+, and, even within this wave of some 200 competitors, I self-seed myself near the back. This Half Ironman swim distance is 1.9km, so I seed myself at around one hour. I am really not confident in open water and don't want others swimming over me or having too many arms and legs thrashing around close to me. After my panicked experience at Snowdonia Slateman, I don't have any high expectations. I just want to be able to get out of the water within the 1 hour 10 minute cut-off.

Standing in the mass line-up for the start, my nerves are kicking in. I want to cry, I'm getting scared, I'm remembering that I have no supporters here, so I'm feeling lost and lonely even amongst such a huge crowd. Beside me is a young girl who seems even more scared than me. She's part of a relay team, and, whilst she's swum in this lake a few times for practice, she is close to tears with fear as well. I find that by chatting to her and reassuring her, I am actually, inwardly, reassuring myself. I share with her how not to go dashing off in the water but take time to get herself settled. This is how I do it (I thought it best not to mention my Slateman panic). For this event, we don't have the opportunity to get acclimatised to the water temperature before the starter horn blows.

It's a continuous roll of people into the water from a floating pontoon. The timing chip on my ankle triggers the bleep of the timing mat. My time has begun. I hit the start button on my watch so I can keep an eye on my timing for each discipline.

Unlike the graceful dives of the athletic bodies of the elites in skintight wetsuits, my entry to the water is more like a baby elephant on ice. The pontoon drops away steeply into the murky lake water that has been churned up by the hundreds of athletes before me. With wobbling legs on the shifting pontoon, there is every chance I will belly-flop into the water. So I choose to take control, sit on my bum and slide in like a big kid. Yes, not graceful, but at least I'm in.

I am so glad I went for the practice swim yesterday; the water feels warm and welcoming. I don't look too far ahead, just to the next buoy and where the kayaks are, for reassurance. As I slowly make my way up the lake, I am conscious of others coming slowly past me. I take a quick glance behind me and all I can see is kayaks. No more pink swim caps behind me; I am last. My heart sinks: 'Oh, no – I'm last, I'm not going to make this!' But then I remember my training. I have to keep focussed and remember how I tackle endurance swims at home: I take time to settle in but actually know I can complete the distance in the time. Today we have 1 hour 10 minutes to complete the swim, and this is within my capabilities. Slowly but surely, everything starts to fall into place. I focus on the pink swim caps in front of me, and, like the hands on a clock, moving forward without you really noticing, I start to catch them. I start to pass a few of the swimmers. Some of them are just slowing down – perhaps they went off too fast to start with? Some of them are even calling for assistance from the kayaks.

As I pass each one, my confidence grows a tiny bit more. Before I know it, I'm at the top of the lake and swimming around the top buoy. Now it's just a straight swim to the slipway. As I sight for each buoy, not only do I find myself passing more pink swim caps, but now there are some blue ones that I'm closing in on. My confidence is now starting to soar – I've actually caught up with the back of the previous wave!

As my fingertips and then my knees touch the slipway, I stumble up to my feet. The sensation of standing makes my head spin, but the volunteers on the waterside help me to steady myself before running to the transition tent, peeling my wetsuit down to my waist as I go. As I exited the water I took a quick glance at my watch – 56 minutes 47 seconds. 'Oh my word!' my brain screams. 'I knew it felt good in the water once I'd relaxed and got going.' I felt as though I was on target, but this put me three minutes ahead of my target time. For a triathlete like me, who finds themselves chasing cut-off times, a saving of three minutes is great.

The transition tent is a whole new experience, and I take time to sit down and dry my feet whilst munching on a banana. I stuff my wetsuit, goggles and cap into my transition bag and drop it with the volunteers as I head out with my helmet and bike shoes on to grab Piston. The weather isn't helping today, as it started raining whilst we were swimming. The forecast for today was not great, so it looks like it's going to be a long, wet slog. With no supporters at this event, it's just me against the clock. I now have 56 miles to ride. Heading out on to the road, the rain gets heavier. Whilst I'm not bothered by rain, it does make the road surface more slippery, so pushing hard going into corners isn't going to happen!

Leaving transition, I've opted to put on a short-sleeve cycle jersey over my wet trisuit. In these first few miles, I am really regretting this, as my arms are so cold. But there's nothing I can do about it now. I will just have to cycle hard to keep warm.

My pace feels good, considering the weather conditions, and the miles of tarmac keep rolling by. I know I am more of a 'back of the pack' rider. I'm not super-fast, but I do have stamina for the endurance. It's important not to overcook it as faster cyclists come past me. I know I can ride 56 miles in the time and still make the cut-off.

Into the last stages of the bike course, and the route starts to climb; a long, long steady climb stretches out in front of me. This doesn't faze me at all, considering I train in hilly north Devon, and I realise I am actually passing cyclists who are pushing their bikes up the hill. All that training at home is paying off. Every direction from my home starts with a hill, some of which are longer or steeper than this one. We're riding up through a residential area, and families are out in their front gardens, clapping and cheering us as we pass. There's no way I'd want to get off and push in front of spectators – that's my motivation to keep the pedals turning.

At the top of the hill, we ride a loop around the top of the Shugborough estate. Grinning from ear to ear, I know it's pretty much all downhill from here to the transition area for the run. This is really happening, this is doable – I am going to get this Half Ironman under my belt!

My transition from bike to run is slower than I had hoped. After making sure to manage my intake of energy

THIRTEEN

bars and the occasional half a banana that I picked up at the feed stations on the way around the bike course, I have so far not needed to stop for the toilet. But now, after being out on the road for over four hours, my stoma is getting active. Any other triathlete may be able to 'hang on', but for me, I can feel the tell-tale bulge of my stoma bag, which forces me to make this extended pit stop at the Portaloo. Not the most salubrious of locations, but a 'baggy' girl's got to do what a 'baggy' girl's got to do!

In the transition tent, I change into my running shoes, feeling more comfortable now that I've sorted my bag out. Running across the uneven grassy route, my legs feel a bit wobbly and not too keen to run. But I'm on track with my timing – well, maybe just a little bit behind now – but knowing how long it will take me to run a half-marathon, I know this is the final leg. It's a three-loop course around the Shugborough estate and out on to the road. As I'd been coming in at the end of the bike course, I'd passed the triathletes who were already on the run. It was still a soggy, wet afternoon, and this run was going to be a slog.

One thing I love about triathlons as a slower competitor is the amazing camaraderie you get from others. We are all battling the same pain, we've all struggled to get here and we all have the same dream. I find myself running alongside a guy called Simon, and we get chatting as we run. We are running at about the same pace, but he is a loop ahead of me. As I start to flag, he tells me to keep going; and likewise, as he starts to flag, I'm there beside him to keep him motivated too. We talk about our times and our pace, knowing we are both going to make it. As we struggle on the climbs, we agree to walk through the feed stations and we stick together. Having been here all weekend feeling alone, this man is a rock for me – someone to tell me to keep pushing.

As we finish the second loop, we have to go our separate ways. He's heading off in the direction of the finishers' chute, wishing me the best of luck and encouraging me to keep pushing on this last loop. I might be closer to the wire than I'd hoped, as the run is turning out to be slower than I had planned. As I pass the top of the chute, I hear the commentator calling out his name and number, and the crowd are cheering him in. As I look over my shoulder, I see his arms raised running down the red carpet; there's a lump in my throat and tears in my eyes. I am so glad to see him finish; now I've just got to dig deep on my own for one last lap, and that will be me!

The course takes me around the back of the manor house, through the gardens. What had been a dusty path is now a muddy, slushy mess with the continuous rain and nearly 2,000 pairs of feet trampling through it. My slow speed means I'm not feeling particularly warm, but I keep moving, putting one foot in front of the other, as the rain continues to fall, knowing I just have to push. Keeping an eye on my watch, I've worked out that at the pace I am doing now I will get in within the final cut-off time. I'm joined by another lady who is pacing herself just to finish. She's running for a charity, and as long as she finishes she will be going out to Kona in Hawaii to race, raising money for her good cause. The thought of going to Kona, the ultimate location for any Ironman competitor, is huge and very exciting.

We push on in the driving rain, now so soaked to the skin that we just don't care. As we run back along the path that had looped around the building, a man steps out in my way. I dart to one side to try to avoid running into him,

THIRTEEN

and he steps to the side as well, blocking my way. 'What is this man doing?' I think to myself. With his hand up in front of me, he's saying, 'I'm very sorry, you've got to stop.'

'Stop? Why are you stopping me?'

'You haven't made the run cut-off. You won't finish today.'

I'm stunned and look at my watch.

'I've still got just over an hour left before the finish line closes, and I've only got 5km left to run.'

The referee stands his ground, assuring me that I've still got over 9km yet to go and I won't make that in an hour. He's wrong. Worried now that my race time is ticking away, I'm shouting at him that I've got over an hour and 5km left to go, pointing at my Garmin, which has my timer on it. This is unfair – he needs to let me go so I can finish.

With his arms spread wide so I cannot pass, he asks me to give him my race number from around my waist. This cannot be happening! I was inside the run cut-off at nine miles, and I keep telling him I'm already on my last loop, showing him the bands I've collected at each circuit. He won't listen – he's just saying, 'I know it's hard to accept, but you haven't made it this time.'

'Haven't made it? You're wrong – you shouldn't be stopping me.'

It's a losing battle. This man will not let me, or the lady I am running with, go any further. The tears are rolling down my face. As the minutes tick by arguing with him, I see my chance at finishing the race slipping away. I can hear the commentator across the field cheering in the competitors as they are crossing the line.

The man takes my bib number from me, and with that I collapse on the ground crying my heart out. I came here to finish my first Ironman event and now I have been cheated out of it by someone who won't listen. He walks away, leaving me sat in the dirt crying my heart out. The lady who is running with me has argued as hard alongside me, and she drifts away to find her friends and family. We all have to deal with this in our own way.

    The rain is cold, and I'm only wearing a sleeveless trisuit. Having stopped running after being out in this atrocious weather for seven hours, my body is cooling down fast and I'm starting to shiver. 'So what do I do now?' I say out loud to no one but myself. Picking myself up off the floor, I look around to get my bearings. My chest hurts from the deep sobbing, which I cannot control. I'm broken; I'm devastated.

    I stumble across the path and have to climb over a fence. I walk towards the top of the finishers' chute, where I see others still enjoying their moment on the red carpet. I cannot bear to watch them. I've no idea what I'm meant to do now. I blindly wander across the field, oblivious to where I am or where I am meant to go to find my clothes. If I had crossed the finish line, then it's all so organised; but just left on the side of the path without instruction, I am lost in the depths of darkness and distress, wandering aimlessly. From out of the blue a spectator comes up to me, clearly concerned. I'm ranting about being unfairly stopped, and she gives me a hug and wraps me in a plastic rain cover to try to help me get warm and keep the rain off. I thank her for her kindness and follow the directions of a marshal towards the finishers' tent, where I am told my white bag has been transported with my day clothes in.

    Inside the tent, triathletes are all congratulating each other, with their Ironman medals hung proudly around their necks. I slump into a hard, plastic chair, staring

THIRTEEN

blankly at the floor, snuffling. My tears of devastation turn quickly to anger at the unfairness of it. I was going to finish. Another competitor, who had been behind us, had spotted what was happening to us and had dodged behind a tree and snuck around the back of the marshal, and that man went on to finish and claim his just reward. I take the cup of hot tea offered by the young girl in the tent and apologise for my ranting.

As I show my race number, tattooed on my arm, the man running the bagging area passes me my white transition bag with my clothes in and directs me to pick up my finisher's T-shirt with a cheery 'Congratulations'. I look daggers at him and snap 'I wasn't allowed to finish. I've been unfairly stopped.' He shrinks back apologetically, and I feel bad that I am snapping the heads off everyone; they don't deserve it – they're the volunteers who give up their time to make this event happen for us.

There's nothing left for me to do. I'm lost, I've no one here to give me a hug and tell me it's OK. It's just me, my anger and my tears. I collect Piston and my transition bag containing all my cycle kit from the T2 area and traipse to the lorry that has brought back our transition bags with our wetsuits in. Laden down with three bags and a heart as heavy as lead, I find my way back to my car in the middle of a vast field of vehicles. Ringing home, I burst into floods of tears again at the sound of my husband's voice. He had been tracking me online and seen that I was on course to finish: the Ironman website predicts your expected finish time based on where you are on the course and the pace at which you are progressing through the cut-off points. He'd seen that I had made it past the last cut-off point with time to spare, and then ... nothing. He'd been watching it for hours realising I hadn't finished, worried what had happened.

After a long, weepy phone call I hang up and sit crying in my car for another hour. I don't know why I'm still sat here, just watching everyone else leaving. What difference is it going to make, just sitting here? I stare at the large solitary tree in the middle of the field in front of me. When I saw this tree this morning in the ridiculously small hours, I had been full of excitement and expectation. Now I'm empty.

Over the next two days, the lady who I had been running with and had also been stopped, made contact with me to say her charity were appealing to the organisers about her being incorrectly stopped, and she had made sure to include my name and race number in their appeal. Within the week, with my own official complaint filed as well, we heard that the incident had been investigated and that we were correct. The referee who had stepped out in front of us had been in the wrong place on the course. He'd been standing on the wrong side of the path, and we shouldn't have been stopped. The organisers gave me the choice of a refund or a replacement entry to the following year's event.

It's one thing proving that you were right, but when it came to this race, what was taken away from me was all those hours of training, all those hours I had sacrificed with my family to get to be in a position to compete and finish. A bit of me didn't want to do this race again, but now I've got the full Ironman at Bolton coming up, I am taking from this experience the fact that I still learned loads. It wasn't just about getting to grips with the split transitions – it was learning what it will take out of me both mentally and physically to compete at Ironman UK. In a way, I have to thank this individual referee for making me look forward and keep pushing the boundaries.

Chapter Fourteen

IN THE last few weeks I've had to take stock of what happened at Staffordshire. I've gone over it again and again in my head, thinking what I could have done differently. In my head, I envisage myself running past the man who stopped me, of handing over my race number and still running on regardless. But it's pointless thinking about what could have been. What would my life have been like if I hadn't had my surgery? I have no doubt that I would never have even considered being a triathlete, and I would never have found so many wonderful, inspiring people through Ostomy Lifestyle Athletes, or such fantastic, supporting friends through the North Devon Tri Club. Things happen in our lives that are out of our control, and that referee at Staffordshire was just another test.

Ironman UK is looming, and I am going to do it. I have trained hard, recovered from injury and come back from some knock-backs. Now I am heading to Bolton to meet Marc Mahoney, who I met through OLA – he lives locally and knows the route. He's going to take me out on the course so I can get a feel for it. I know this bike route has a couple of big, big climbs which are notorious, so I want to tackle them before race day so that I am mentally prepared.

Outside the B&B where I am staying, I am getting Piston ready for our ride, when Marc rides in. It's bizarre to meet someone for the first time face-to-face when you feel you've already known them a lifetime. Marc's had surgery too, and it's great to be able to talk openly about how we got to this point with our stomas. Marc's a keen cyclist, and I am so grateful that he can lead me out around the course. We're not starting from where it will begin on race day, but we are still going to do one loop. On race day, I am going to have to ride two loops, which means climbing the monster hills – Sheephouse Lane and Hunters Hill – twice. These are going to be the killers for me.

Our day is peppered with rain showers and sunshine. Whilst Marc makes the hills look relatively easy, I slog away at them, accepting that at some point I am going to have to get off the bike and walk. I may not be exactly enjoying this ride, because of the climbs and the dawning realisation of what I have taken on, but I am so glad I made the effort to come up here a couple of weeks earlier to see it first-hand.

*****

On Saturday morning, I've worked out a tight schedule for getting racked up and having a practice swim in the lake. However, this time I also have to plan in some time with Damian and the film crew. They have worked with both Trio Ostomy Care and Vanilla Blush before, and today Nicola Dames of Vanilla Blush is going to be joining us for the first time – she'd like to do some photography shoots together, as I am now going to be wearing a fantastic trisuit she's had designed for me for Ironman. Hanging

FOURTEEN

about in the car park, I soon catch up with Damian and Nicola. However, they're being really cagey. From behind me I hear 'Hello' in a soft Dutch voice ... I cannot believe it, Mark Vos, another OLA elite cyclist who I have never had the pleasure of meeting, but speak to all the time, has turned up on his bike with Marc Mahoney. The whole group were in cahoots together to surprise me. Not only that, but they've made some massive banners to wave on the roadside. They've just blown me away!

We spend a couple of hours chilling out with some photography and interviews to camera for Vanilla Blush before I can rack up Piston in the most enormous caged transition area. It's boggy underfoot from all the recent rain, and I'm nervous leaving Piston out overnight, but I am getting more accustomed to the split transitions and am better prepared with my transition bike bag this time.

After a practice swim in Pennington Flash, I am feeling ready. Saying farewell to my supporters, I drive to the Macron Stadium, where Transition Two and the finish line are. Leaving my run bag hanging on its peg, I walk through the transition area so I know where I am going to be dropping off Piston, and make sure I know the route through the tent and out on to the run. This will be my first marathon. I've trained for this and know it will be both physically and mentally tough, but I am going to give it my best shot. Based on the time I should have crossed the line at Staffordshire 70.3, if I'd not been stopped, I reckon I am going to cross the line inside the final time. It might be close, but I'm going to do it.

Athletes are called into the stadium for the race briefing. It's huge! The number of competitors in this one enormous room is beyond belief. There's a buzz of excitement as the lights drop and the stage is lit. This race briefing is more like a show, one that is going to fire us all up and drive us to fulfil our ambition of being an Ironman. Sitting at the table surrounded by avid competitors listening to details of the course, I'm struck by the sight on stage of the man who had stopped me at Staffordshire. I thought I was over this, the issue was resolved and I'd moved on. But here and now, all that heartache and anger wells back up inside me. If anything is going to put a fire in my belly to prove a point tomorrow, this is it.

* * * * *

Sunday morning comes around quickly; it's difficult trying to fall asleep at 9pm knowing you've got to be up at 3am. The hotel is laying on breakfast for the athletes who are staying here, but wandering into the restaurant area I can see it's decidedly lacking. I didn't expect a full cooked breakfast or anything like that to be laid on, but I usually start the day with porridge and bananas before a race. All that we've got to choose from are small packets of breakfast cereal, toast and cold croissants. There's nothing nutritious in this lot – it's just a feeble attempt at a continental breakfast. How on earth will this sustain the competitors? My body isn't really feeling hungry at this unearthly hour, but I force myself to eat some cereal and toast. I've got my own bars packed in my bag, as well as bananas, so that will have to do for topping me up.

Driving down to the finish line in Bolton to leave my car, the silence of the roads has a surreal feel to it, especially in an area like this that you would expect to be a hive of activity. With the hundreds of other competitors, I take the bus to the swim start and begin my ritual of preparing for the race. It's rained again overnight, and the transition area is a quagmire. As I check the bike and eat a banana,

FOURTEEN

my toes squelch through mud on to the matted area that lines the route down to the water's edge. This race has a rolling start, whereby as the horn goes, the competitors at the front will start. Every competitor's time will only start when their timing chip crosses the mat as they enter the water. Again we have to self-seed ourselves, based on how long we expect to take in the swim. I'm near the back at 2 hours. The total time allowed for the swim is 2 hours 20 minutes. I've hedged my bets a bit on my timing, as I've never swum this distance in open water before.

It takes half an hour for me to reach the starting mat, but it's a relief to finally get in the water – all the waiting just messes with your head. The swim is 2.4 miles and is two laps of the lake. The elite swimmers in their gold caps have gone out first. As I swim up the first stretch of open water, getting my rhythm, I can hear splashing behind me. A glance back and I can see the elite group coming towards me – fast! Whilst I'm just heading out on my first loop, these guys are on their second lap. I hold my nerve and remember that these swimmers don't want to swim over me because I would slow them down. If I stay in a straight line, I will be clearly visible. My thinking pays off as the gold caps swim left and right of me at a blistering pace, sending the water into a frenzy around me. Hold your nerve, hold your nerve. They're past and I can relax again.

The swim goes well, and before I know it I'm taking the last few strokes towards the pontoon out of the water. I get to my feet and run along the matting, with the crowds crammed up against the side cheering on all the competitors. My watch shows me I've just been around the first lap in just over 45 minutes; that's a personal best. I cannot miss the green and white North Devon Tri Club jackets of Donna Marriott and Tina Kiff-Jamieson, who have both come out to support me today. High-fiving them as I go, I am elated. I jump back into the water, and I'm out on the second loop. 'I've done one loop, so this is easy now,' I tell myself. It's always great to get past the halfway mark. Around the top two buoys, and I am cutting through the water, passing swimmer after swimmer. This feels fantastic.

Suddenly I feel a pain shooting through my left calf. Cramp! As I try to shake it out, my right leg cramps up too. The pain in both legs is beyond belief. Please, not now.

'Help! help!'

There are no kayaks anywhere near me, and I am having to tread water.

'Help! Please help!' I sob as loudly as I can, panic rising. The kayaks simply cannot hear me.

Suddenly there's a burst of activity around me: two competitors are swimming to me at speed. As they reach me, I explain my legs have both cramped up. Whilst one of the men swims forward and shouts for the attention of a kayak, the other stays with me, holding my arm in reassurance until the boat can get to me. As the kayak arrives, I tell him to keep pushing on. I am overwhelmed at the kindness of these two men: men who, like me, are near the back, but yet they have jeopordised their dream of being an Ironman to come to my assistance without a second thought. I found out later that at least one of them went on to finish.

After what feels like an eternity holding on to the kayak, the cramping in my legs subsides and I'm able to swim again, albeit somewhat slower. It's a relief to reach the shore to the cheers of Donna and Tina. I've completed

FOURTEEN

the swim in 1 hour 45 minutes despite my hold-up – way faster than I had imagined.

I run into the transition tent, peeling off my wetsuit and swim cap as I go. Changing into my bike shoes, I'm going to have to use the Portaloo. My stoma bag is filling up; usually the porridge and bananas is enough to settle it until well into the bike stage, but with just cereal for breakfast, this has caused me a lot more problems. The toilet stop adds more minutes on to my time, but, being happy with my swim time, I'm not too concerned. What concerns me more is my calf muscles, which are still feeling sore from the cramp.

I know I have to eat and replenish the fuel stores in my body. As I mount the bike out of transition, I make sure to eat a banana as a quick fuel top-up. I'm glad I did the ride around the course a few weeks ago with Marc, as it's all feeling familiar. I know what the terrain is going to be like for a while before I have to face the first of the hills. That's not to say there aren't other hills to tackle, but they're not as long.

Riding the course, it feels like you're competing in the Tour de France. The roadside support is out of this world. At every town, the streets are lined with cheering supporters, there are street parties and people in fancy dress everywhere, and children with home-made banners.

As I come to a short hill climb along a street lined with spectators, I get an overwhelming feeling of being sick. I cannot let this happen here, or anywhere for that matter. My body needs to conserve fuel, not get rid of it. Plus, there is no way I can possibly get off the bike and push it up this hill in front of all these people. I dig deep, pinning a smile on my face as I ride through the crowds, just hoping and praying that there isn't another hill around the next corner. I recognise that the sickness feeling is due to lack of food; I've not eaten enough breakfast for the swim and my body is depleted. I've got to get past this feeling and keep eating and drinking my electrolyte drink, no matter what.

The biggest hill is the 3km-long Sheephouse Lane, with a gradient of 22%. This is the one that was beating me on my ride out with Marc. As I hit the bottom of the hill, I can hear shrieking: 'Come on Caroline. Come on!' Nicola Dames is stood on the side of the road with not only Marc Mahoney and Mark Vos, but a number of other ostomy athletes including Jason Podger and Christel Carr-Elliott. After recovering from her hit-and-run accident, Christel had come to cheer me on as part of her UK tour, having flown in from the USA. Just as I was flagging at the sight of the hill before me, this amazing bunch of people gave me the injection of determination to get out of the saddle and go full-on into the hill. At the top of the hill is a treat: the infamous Sheephouse Lane Fancy Dress Party, a bunch of masked musclemen who play loud music, wave banners with words of encouragement and are all-round motivators.

The technical descent is the time to let Piston fly, and I love the freedom. On the flat, the crowds are cheering, and I can see the female champion, Lucy Gossage, coming by me as she's coming round on her second loop.

I know from the feel of my legs that I'm not riding at the pace I should be, and I'm calculating where I am on the course compared with my time. There are two cut-offs on this bike route, one at around 60 miles and the other around 81 miles. I know I've gone through the first one, albeit a lot closer than I'd planned, so I push hard to hit the second one. Looking at my watch, it's touch and go

FOURTEEN

whether I made it through in time. There's no one around at that point, so I decide I have to make the assumption that I'm through and keep pushing.

I'm on to the second loop, and yet again I am confronting Sheephouse Lane. This time, however, I am struggling. I've not been keeping on top of my fuel, as I'm feeling sick again and struggled to swallow it down, so I know my body is rebelling. I'm determined to push through, though, no matter what. As the climb gets steeper, my legs won't turn the pedals, and I resort to getting off and pushing. Walking uphill in cleats pulls on your calf muscles, and I lean into the handlebars to push Piston up this hill.

Along the roadside, Jason and Christel are still waiting to cheer me on, whilst the others have headed to the transition area to see me come in. My legs are like lead, the road feels steeper than last time and I can hear the engine of the sweeper van ticking along behind me. I've done the numbers in my head. There's only half an hour until the cut-off at Transition Two and I've still got 17 miles to ride, including climbing this hill. Even if I was at the top, I'd never be able to make it in time. The van pulls up alongside me; with the window wound down, the driver says to me, 'You know what I'm about to say, don't you?'

With that, I stop pushing. I admit defeat. I'm not going to be an Ironman. I'm thankful that Jason and Christel are there with me as I put the bike down in the grass and cry.

* * * * *

After a month of rest from Ironman, I feel ready to pick up where I left off, but at a much gentler pace. My family have put up with weekends of me being out on the bike or out early in the mornings training. I've tried my best not to let it impact on the time I have with my family and work, but it does definitely mean a lot of sacrifices. As races have always been on a Sunday, and are generally a long way from north Devon, Craig and the children have not been able to come up and watch me race. But I have recruited them into being my sub-coaches, to feel a part of my journey, especially as the training commitment gets heavier towards Ironman. I put a copy of my Training Peaks plan up on the wall in the kitchen. On here I've mapped out all the training sessions I have to do in a week. The children can then see my statistics from each swim, bike or run, and fill them in on the chart. But they've also been given permission to nag me to go out. Often after school Robert or Natasha ask, 'Mum, did you run this morning?' If I confess I haven't, they will make sure I go out after dinner to get it done.

Now I have to regroup and think what I want to do from here. Upon reflection, I know I messed up with the nutrition. I didn't approach it like another discipline, and that poor breakfast on race day had definitely put me on the start of a slippery slope for the rest of the day. James has been a fantastic coach, and he's got me this far. I could never have attempted these Ironman events this year without his coaching, but I now need to look at what else I need to do to improve. It's not just about the physical training.

I first met Simon de Burgh of Tri Force Endurance when I was on the exhibition stand at Tri Expo in Manchester earlier in the year. In those two days spent with him, I came to see not only the geekiness of understanding your nutrition, but that this man not only knows it, he has actually finished Ironman events himself. He really puts

FOURTEEN

his knowledge into practice for himself and his clients. So I share with him where I am at with my training, my year of DNFs (Did Not Finish) and also about my ileostomy.

Maybe he sees me as a new challenge, but he seems as excited at the prospect of working with me as I do with him. I've also had confirmation from Reena at Trio Ostomy Care that they would like to continue sponsoring me into 2017 as my exclusive sponsor, rather than being part of a dual sponsorship arrangement as they were last year. Things are falling into place wonderfully. I have the bike, but now I can afford to hire Simon and Billy Harris from Tri Force Endurance to coach me to the next level. We start with some one-to-one sessions so that Simon can assess my abilities. In the pool, he watches my technique and makes some immediate tweaks. He also starts planning my training, gradually increasing my distances in the pool as well as the technical aspects.

Combined with this, he's really understanding my family lifestyle and ensuring that the plan he is setting for me actually works around my other commitments. There's no point in setting training sessions for me that I am simply not going to be able to get done. His approach is far more holistic, and it's working great. I am achieving more training, but at the same time I am gaining all the additional knowledge about nutrition. I am not just eating better, but eating smarter and understanding how the food we eat fuels our body, together with relevant supplements.

Having discussed what worked and what didn't work in 2016, the plan for 2017 is to go back to Ironman Staffordshire 70.3 and nail it. I'm not to fill my schedule with loads of other big races, but to remain focussed on my goal. Let's do this.

LOO ROLLS TO LYCRA

* * * * *

There are times when I feel 'normal' and I forget I have a stoma. That's a good thing, because I don't allow it to hold me back in any way. However, from time to time it can kick back.

In the early days of having my ileostomy, I was very conscious, when driving, of the seat belt being pulled across my stoma bag; it sits at just the wrong point and can be uncomfortable on long journeys. I drive a great deal for work and meetings, and on one particular summer's day I'm driving up the M5 for a meeting, with an overnight stay in a hotel.

My drive up the motorway has been a pretty clear run all day and I'm making good time, but having passed a couple of service stations, ignoring that little niggle in the back of my mind that I ought to stop for a toilet break, I begin to feel the burning sensation around my stoma. Knowing that this acidic burn means the output is getting under my flange and on to my skin, it's essential that I stop at the next services.

As Bridgewater Services come into view, I peel off and head for the car park.

These particular services don't have one of those big, open expanses of car parking, but a multi-storey car park that is a short walk away from the entrance to the service station itself across a parking area for motorcycles and large vehicles that won't fit in the multi-storey. Finding a space on the ground floor, I park the large jeep-style courtesy car that I have today in a parking bay and grab my rucksack. The burning on my skin is getting worse, and I know that if I don't change this bag soon it could be disastrous.

FOURTEEN

In the ladies' toilets, I dash into a cubicle. I don't usually bother with using the disabled toilet facilities unless I really need to, so, dropping my rucksack on the floor, it's routine for me to be able to peel off my bag and do a quick change – although it would be a darn site easier if there was a toilet seat or something to lay all my stoma kit out on.

As I lift my T-shirt and turn down the top of my trousers, disaster strikes. The reason the burning on my skin was so bad is because, now that I have stood up from driving, the flange has given out completely. The poo output in my bag has managed to get out completely from under the flange and has gone everywhere! It's like an explosion in my trousers!

I step out of my trousers, which have some mess on them and will need rinsing out, but my knickers have completely had it! Thankfully, wearing some high-waisted knickers today has helped to contain the explosion. I've no option but to roll up the knickers in some toilet paper and dispose of them in the personal hygiene bin. Stripped from the waist down, I can now take off the stoma bag that is hanging off my abdomen and clean myself up. I have an emergency kit in my rucksack at all times with spare stoma bags and wipes, so at least I can tidy myself up and put on a clean bag.

Round one complete, the next dilemma is: what do I do now? I cannot put my trousers back on as they're covered in poo! My knickers are in the bin and I'm stood in a small toilet cubicle in a service station with a male cleaning attendant wandering about! I have to at least get out to the hand basins to rinse my trousers out, but how on earth am I going to do that with nothing on! My brain is frozen. There's no way out of here! I spot my sweatshirt sitting on top of my rucksack. Miracle: I can wear that. Tying it around my waist is useless – either my backside is exposed, or my front. I know, I can wear it like a pair of trousers. I step into one arm, but as I try to get the other leg in down the second arm, it's clear this isn't going to work either. There's nothing left to do but make a mad dash to the sink half-naked and hope no one sees me. Hold on – maybe I could mummify myself from my waist down, I think, as I grab at the half-full toilet roll hanging on its roller. Nope, that would just fall off the moment I move.

    I rummage around in my rucksack, wishing it was like something out of Harry Potter where anything you need comes out. My hand finds something soft at the bottom of the bag. Spare knickers? Pulling the material out, my heart sinks. It's not knickers – it's my Outlaw triathlon neck buff. Pulling at the material, thinking laterally, I've got only one last idea. I stretch the buff wide and step my left leg in; pulling it wider still, I put my right leg in. So far, so good! With some further stretching and wiggling I manage to get the buff up over my bum. I cannot believe my luck. It might be the skimpiest of skirts ever known to man, but it covers all the essential areas. Letting my T-shirt drop down over the top, around my waist, who would know that this wasn't a skirt?

    Knowing that I have a whole suitcase full of clothes in the back of the courtesy car, I gingerly walk out of the service station. As I mince my way with pigeon-toed steps past the police car that is now sitting outside, I must look like the biggest tart in town. Relieved to get to the car, I blip the button to unlock it, only for all the alarms to go off. Talk about calling attention to yourself! After a hurried phone call to the garage, they thankfully manage to give me instructions on how to turn off the alarm

FOURTEEN

system before I have the police coming over to investigate further.

My lesson was learned; never go out without spare knickers!

Chapter Fifteen

IT'S BEEN a long journey getting back to Ironman Staffordshire both physically and mentally. In order to race this weekend, I've had to make some sacrifices (yet again). With my husband having to work evening shifts, I've had to call upon favours with my neighbour to come and babysit the children from teatime on Friday until Craig gets in from work at 10pm. I couldn't switch into 'athlete mode' today, when I know other competitors would have all been registering knowing they can be really relaxed tomorrow, Saturday, for setting up. For me, I am still being mum. My first role is to be there for my children, and I need to be at home when they get in from school, put the school uniforms on to wash and make them their tea, before I can start loading the car.

After double-checking my suitcase and my tri bag yet again, ensuring I have remembered everything, I can load up the car. Lifting Piston up on to the roof is like putting her up on to a pedestal – my flag. I'm a cyclist, I'm a triathlete.

Hugs and kisses with the children, I wave out of the car window as I drive off; this is now my big adventure. This

FIFTEEN

is me. This is Caroline the triathlete who has unfinished business to deal with.

As I arrive on site at Shugborough Hall before 8am on Saturday, to prepare myself for race day tomorrow, I'm hit with a sudden wave of emotion. I've only ever been here once before, and yet it all seems so familiar. The long, winding roadway that meanders down towards where the giant marquees are set up, waiting for a couple of thousand wannabe Ironmen and women to bring the place to life.

Across the empty field that will tomorrow be filled with cars, amongst the dots of men and women in hi-viz jackets, I spot the classic folly, half-hidden amongst the trees, that was one of my visual markers for where I parked my car last year. In the centre of the field across to my right is a large, sprawling tree – the tree that I parked beside in my car last year and cried and cried. My chest tightens and tears roll gently down my face as I scan the scene, transporting me back 12 months. The emotion of last year is as raw now as if it had just happened. At the end of the road in front of me, I can see the large, white Transition Two marquee, with its caged outdoor arena just waiting for over 2,000 bicycles to be racked up at speed tomorrow in the heat of the event.

On the radio, Frankie Valli and the Four Seasons are singing 'Big Girls Don't Cry'. I laugh out loud at the irony of the song as I'm sat here in my car with tear stains on my face. 'Oh yes, they do!' I say back to the invisible crooner on the radio … 'Oh yes, they do!'

Straight ahead I see the Athletes' Village – two long, large marquees, propped up with ropes and poles like surreal elongated circus tents, surrounding the finishers' chute to that classically recognisable red carpet and finish line! The registration tent houses the triathlon expo, where you can spend an absolute fortune on branded Ironman merchandise. They are a smart organisation and know exactly how to leverage additional earnings from the eager triathletes who are keen to demonstrate their prowess on the course tomorrow. Branded caps, mugs and teddy bears, and then the plethora of T-shirts, running kit and hoodies with the M-Dot Ironman logo on the back, made up of all the names of the competitors. Of course, every competitor wants a T-shirt with their name on, but for me the only T-shirt I've got my eye on is the Finisher's T-shirt that will be legitimately given to me after I cross that finish line.

I learned a lot from my experience last year, and I'm feeling more relaxed today. I am eternally grateful to my friend and fellow competitor Pete Gough, for picking up my car-parking pass yesterday, thus saving me anxiety of trying to pick it up on Saturday morning from the centre of Stafford. I enter the expo tent with clear plans for how to get set up today, with the two separate transition areas 20 miles apart. I head through the exhibition stands, blinkered to all the great products on display, to get my registration done as quickly as possible.

The volunteers at Ironman events are some of the most amazing people – they will have been on site for several days for hours and hours to get this whole show running like clockwork. Familiar faces are there year after year, and I know they do it for us, to help us be the best we can be. Collecting my registration pack, I couldn't resist a quick hug with Iron-mums Linda Ogden and Janet Gibson, who have followed my journey and live the ups and downs with us.

I head over in the car to Chasewater, planning to get a practice swim in the lake. This is the start and Transition

FIFTEEN

One, so I take the opportunity to rack Piston up in the fenced transition area and get my bearings of where my bike is located, so I can find it quickly in the race. Déjà vu is overwhelming, taking me back to the anxiety of setting up last year. Considering this race is in June and last year I ran it in pouring rain, the weather this year has been unbearably and unseasonably hot these last two days, and tomorrow is not going to be any different. This raises issues with tyres – I have seen tyres pop in extreme weather, and, with my bike having to be out here all day today in sweltering temperatures, I cannot risk turning up tomorrow and finding my tyres have blown up. I let some air pressure out of the tyres – tomorrow morning I can top them up with a track pump before the race starts.

After dropping my T1 bike bag into the transition tent, containing my helmet, race shoes, race belt with my bib number on it, my energy bars, a towel and talc, I head over to the lakeside. This year I've not had any opportunity for open-water swim practice, so it was crucial for me to get to this practice session. I know I can swim and I know I can do this distance in this lake, but it's the psychological proof I need to give myself by getting in and swimming part of the course.

Having only just picked up my new sponsor's trisuit two days ago, I've not had an opportunity to do any training in it, so I decide to wear this under my wetsuit so I can get the feel of it for tomorrow. It's like a second skin – beautifully fine material that will dry quickly when I'm out on the bike course. I pull on my old second-hand wetsuit that I've had since I started triathlon; it's definitely showing its age, with fingernail punctures here and there, and it's not really the best-fitting wetsuit, but it does the job. I bought it as an ex-demo wetsuit originally, and it's lasted well, but it's probably not quite up to scratch with the rest of my kit now. I swim up the lake and around one of the marker buoys, and head back to where we will exit the water tomorrow. It feels good to be back in the lake. Let's hope I can improve on my time from last year of just under 57 minutes.

Sitting out beside the water, warming myself in the sun after changing back into my shorts and T-shirt, I cannot believe how relaxed I'm feeling with the whole event today. I know what's to come tomorrow, I know what I have to do today to get set up, and I'm feeling just fine with it all.

I make a final check of my T1 bike bag – believe me, I empty and refill that bag several times, talking out loud to myself, to make sure I've not forgotten anything. At some point you just have to tell yourself to leave it alone, everything is there, and just walk away from it! A final check on the bike, and I leave the transition area and head back to Shugborough to go through the whole process again with my run bag in Transition Two: shoes, hat, gels, banana… spare stoma kit! In the excitement of setting up for triathlon, I have to make sure that, both on the bike and on the run, I have my emergency stoma bag kit, just in case I have to make a bag change. Not something your average triathlete has to consider! This usually means my transition times can be longer than average too, with a dash to the Portaloo.

Keeping myself out of the sun and resting up as best I can, I wait patiently for the minutes to tick by until the race briefing. Looking at the finish line, with its tiered seating along the red carpet, up to the big, iconic finish-line gantry with the giant digital clock above it, I contemplate what tomorrow will bring. Here, right in front of me, is my dream: to run down that carpet and

FIFTEEN

cross that line and put right the wrongs that were done to me last year. I can only do my best, but I am going to push as hard as I can to make sure there is no repeat of last year.

My mobile phone rings, bringing me back to the present. It's my coach, Simon. He's checking firstly that I am not outside in the sun, dehydrating. 'No, coach,' I say with a big smile, 'I'm sat in the briefing tent with my feet up, and I've been drinking all day with electrolytes in my water bottle.'

'Good,' he says. 'Stay on it and make sure you rest as much as possible today, and tomorrow you stick to the food and drink plan that you've practised. It's crucial you stay hydrated, as it's going to be hot out there tomorrow.'

It's great to hear his voice … final race checks, final instructions and a real pep talk! Focus, focus, focus. This is my A race with lots to prove. I'm here as a triathlete and I need to put aside all thoughts of the stresses and struggles I've been through recently and just keep one vision in mind: to cross that finish line. Simon reminds me to push hard on the swim and remember my race pace from training; on the bike, don't go out too fast, but stick to my race pace – push hard where I can, but don't overcook it. The run in this heat is going to get to everyone, so I need to be well hydrated on the bike, ready for the run. I hang up, knowing that he and Billy, the other coach in my team from Tri Force Endurance, will be here tomorrow to watch and cheer me on.

The race briefing tent is full as the loud music starts up and the Ironman team start to talk through the course and the rules. I've read the pack, and, having been here before, I know what's expected, but it's good to hear it all again. The head referee stands up to talk about cut-offs and the rules about when they will cut people if you don't reach certain points on the course. I bite the inside of my mouth – I will be checking those run cut-offs, and if anyone dares to try to stop me this year, there's going to be hell to pay.

The air in the tent is palpable – a marquee full of (primarily) testosterone. Some will have last-minute jitters, some will be just absorbing all the information. But for sure, every single person in that tent is tingling with excitement. This is the last time we will be sitting down casually before the race. This is the final briefing. After this, we are all on our own out there on the course.

Last year I was confronting this event completely alone, but this year I've got fellow North Devon Tri Club members Brian Mulholland and Susan Standford also racing. We will all be focussing on our own pace and chasing our own targets, but we will also be seeing each other at the start tomorrow.

Race day begins very early. Brian and I have decided to drive to Chasewater, leave my car in the car park there and take our chances on getting back to it at the end of the day. This saves the extra-early start that we would have needed had we decided to take the car to Shugborough first and then take the 40-minute bus journey back to Chasewater. Getting up at 4.30am is early enough! As the elite triathletes start their race at 7am, every competitor, no matter what time your wave start time is, has to be out of the Transition One area for final checks before 6.50am.

As we drive along in the morning light from the hotel, all seems calm and serene. The early-morning light is starting to creep up, but the world is not yet awake. Except, that is, for 2,000 triathletes and the hundreds of marshals and volunteers who make this whole event

FIFTEEN

happen. Without the car park attendants, the bus drivers, the roadside marshals, the kayaks and the volunteers on feed stations, we could not be the athletes we are. The volunteers are our superstars.

As we near the car park, we see an increasing number of athletes walking towards the buses that will take us to Chasewater. They are talking in hushed tones to match the muted light, their white transition bags slung over the shoulder, into which we will each put our daytime clothes – the clothes we will need when we get to the finish line. We park up and join the queue to hop on to the next bus for the short journey to Chasewater. There's a great sense of camaraderie amongst triathletes, and never more so than when they are all seated quietly together on a bus at 6am! Everyone has done all they can to get to this point; now the inevitable will happen. We will race one another for several hours.

In the fenced transition area, I take time to check Piston over. There's a huge hawkmoth resting on my front wheel. Does this mean I'm going to have wings out on the course today? Thankfully my tyres are still in one piece – no bursts. The competitor across from me lends me his track pump, and I reinflate Piston's tyres to a psi level that will give me a fast ride in this dry weather.

Scanning the area, I see fellow Tri Force Endurance athlete Louise Simm. Louise and I are both coached by Simon and Billy, and had never met face-to-face until yesterday at registration. Tri Force Endurance has been an amazingly supportive coaching team and has a closed Facebook group where all their athletes receive lots of extra valuable learning on nutrition and racing, and where we can all share experiences. This online support has been the backbone to my training. Whilst out on the roads alone, I know the rest of the Tri Force team will be watching every step of the way.

Louise and I spot Simon and Billy on the outside of the fence. Like two caged animals, we're pacing around waiting for the start of the race whilst our coaches throw titbits of advice and support through the small wire squares. There are no more little nuggets they can feed us that would make any more difference today. What we have absorbed up until now will have to sustain us around the course.

As the elite triathletes line up to start their race, every other competitor waits anxiously along the edge of the lake, knowing it will shortly be their turn. Brian, Susan and I are all in the last wave together in the 50+ group, so there is a lengthy wait of nearly an hour and a half before it's our turn to get in the lake. Final preparations of toilet-queuing and bagging up my day clothes are the only things left to do. Realising that the truck that takes the white transition bags with my clothes back to the finish is about to leave, I have a last-minute panic that my clothes won't get there. I'm not alone, as another competitor and I rapidly strip under a tree and unceremoniously shove clothes into the tie-top bag. My faithful K-Y Jelly is rubbed up and down my arms and legs, whilst bodyglide is lavishly rubbed around my neck to stop chaffing from my wetsuit. At 8.15am, the heat is already rising, and the organisers keeping tannoying that competitors should keep their wetsuits down to their waist until they are heading on to the pontoon, such is the temperature today.

We are called to line up and seed ourselves along the bank. Last year I expected to do this in an hour and managed to knock three minutes off that, so this year I seed myself around 50 minutes: I might as well aim high.

FIFTEEN

I'm not so terrified this year. Slowly but surely we creep along the pontoon, watching the younger age group riders heading out on their bikes as we are yet to start. Better prepared for the instability of the pontoon this year, I gingerly walk down into the water, lapping up the plastic panels of the pontoon. The bleep of my timing chip crossing the start mat is loud and clear; hitting the start button on my Garmin, I launch myself forward into the water with a splash. The water is warm, like a bath in fact. As I take the first strokes, I feel the trickle of warm water creeping in down the neck of my wetsuit, like a gentle finger being drawn down my back.

This time I am surrounded by swimmers, no longer the backmarker. My face is quickly down in the water, and my breathing technique is rolling nicely. I've switched from breathing every third stroke to breathing every second stroke, as I get more glide on every pull of my arm. It's paying off as I cut a line through the water. The outward swim always seems long, but once around the top buoys I am clearly focussed on the exit. In the early-morning heat, the water was a cool relief, but now I'm up and out along the transition run from the water's edge to the transition tent.

As fast as I can, I peel off my wetsuit, like shedding an old skin; and out emerges the new me, the triathlete me, in a trisuit displaying a vibrant pink galaxy. Proud of who I am and who I ride for, I grab Piston from the rack and run out to the mount line. This year, there's cheering from Simon and Billy as I head out on to the road. A glance at my watch tells me I've smashed a personal best in the swim at 52 minutes!

Having ridden this course last year, and come up for a recce ride with some other ostomates, who are also racing this year, I know what is to come. I love this course, with its undulating roads; I love that it loops around so you pass riders coming the other way, who all cheer each other on; I love the volunteers and the roadside support from all the locals. Brian and Susan are both ahead of me, as are Marc Mahoney, Andy Jamison, Pete Gough and Mark Vos, from Ostomy Lifestyle Athletes, who all have a stoma like me and signed up to Ironman after cheering me on at Ironman UK in Bolton last year.

On the long climb up to the top of Shugborough, I'm dancing in and out of the saddle to make it to the top without getting off, knowing that every person walking up is going to be behind me when I cross that finish line. The long descent back down creates a welcome cool breeze, as temperatures are topping 30°C today.

My Portaloo stop at Transition Two is essential for a quick bag change. I am bang on target with my pace on the bike and can afford a few extra minutes to make sure I've got a fresh bag on, as the sweat on my body could be the undoing of me. Fresh silicone flanges ensure I've got good adhesion, and I rush through to the transition tent for my running shoes.

I've been on the course for five hours, and the sun is belting down – there's no let-up today from the heat. I've drunk more fluids with electrolyte than usual, because I know this heat will dehydrate me rapidly. Throughout the bike route, I was on point, with drinking every 10 to 15 minutes and having a bite of my home-made energy bars every 20 minutes. I practised my nutrition and hydration plans in training, and today it's all proving to be the best thing I could have done. If I don't fuel up right, the training will all have been for nothing.

The run is gruelling in the heat. As I exit the transition tent, the course begins by running around the

FIFTEEN

Shugborough estate: that sodden, muddy path that saw me crumple in despair last year. This year, it's a dusty path, with spectators strung out on either side, cheering on family and friends. Simon and Billy are there! I see them on the side of the path, cheering as they see my intergalactic trisuit coming into view. My legs are like jelly from the bike, but I won't be seen walking (at least where there are spectators). High-fives are a boost as I head out to pick up ice cubes from the volunteers, to rub around my neck. I'm struggling with the heat, but keep drinking the electrolyte drinks that are handed out at the numerous feed stations. On the course, the organisers have set up a number of sprinkler systems for us to run through to keep cool. This mist is cooling momentarily, but nothing can beat the support of the locals.

Running up the roads, there are families having street parties, sat out in the sunshine cheering on the competitors. House after house have rigged up their garden hoses and spray us down as we go through. Children with buckets of cold water and jugs participate, as I run towards them, taking my cap off and asking them to pour it over my head. Group after group, street after street, the public help to keep us cool.

After the second loop, I pass the top of the finishers' chute. Watching competitors running down that red carpet, my heart beats harder, remembering the feeling I had at this point last year, expecting to go on and finish. I see in front of me the nine-mile marker – the final cut-off point – that one single point on this whole course that I want to see. Beside the marker is a feed station, handing out cola, electrolyte, water and ice to put under your hat. In order to beat this cut-off mark, I had to be here by 4.10pm. By my reckoning, I'm well inside this. To be sure,

I shout out to the drink station to ask what the time is, to be told it's 3.45pm. Yes! Yes! Yes! I'm well inside it!

Dragging myself around the back of the manor house for the final time, I come out on to the final stretch of the dusty path: that ominous spot where I was stopped last year. There's no marshal in sight, but my heart beats fast. I want to get through here as fast as I can, so there's absolutely no way I can be stopped.

As I tap along at a steady pace, Simon appears beside me, running along the grass verge in his socks.

'Caroline, you've got to pick the pace up,' he calls out. 'You've only got 50 minutes until the finish cut-off.'

I look at him, shocked – I thought I was doing OK. Where did I go wrong with my calculations? My head is swimming.

'You've got to get round this last loop with no walking, Caroline. You've got to push through and run it all – absolutely no walking. You don't want to miss the cut-off.'

Feeling gutted that I am about to mess this up, I pick up the pace, even though the heat is sapping me. Until now I'd had a run/walk strategy planned – even though I had done more walking at the start of this stage than I had planned. As I hit the road section with its hilly climbs, I resort to power-walking on the uphill sections. My body just cannot run, but I cannot fail. I take on more electrolyte drink and half a banana, and even resort to taking gels to give me that last surge of energy.

From the roads strewn with people cheering us round, I cross into the last trail section, pushing hard where I can and power-walking as fast as I can when I cannot run. On the final path out of the woodland area, I can hear the sound of the commentator calling out names and race numbers, across the fields. I'm close, but I'm not there

FIFTEEN

yet. With half a mile to go until I re-enter the grounds, I make the final right turn. I've been passing competitors walking back with their bikes and medals all along this path, their cheery calls of 'Well done, keep going' ringing in my ears. I still might not make this.

At the turn is a marshal; my heart is thumping so hard. I ask him, 'How long have I got until it closes? I know I'm close.'

'Don't worry, love,' he says, 'you've got at least half an hour still in hand. You'll make it.'

Half an hour!! Half an hour!!

I'm just minutes away from that final path to the finishers' chute and I've got half an hour! The numbers are not stacking up in my head. Simon's got it wrong. There's no way I've just run that loop in 20 minutes.

I turn on to the path on my way towards the chute. Simon and Billy are nowhere to be seen on the path. Choking back the tears, I filter into the top of the tunnel, grinning like a Cheshire cat. Before me is that iconic red carpet with the Ironman gantry at the end. Pumping the air, I've made it to the top of the red carpet. I hear the commentator's voice: 'She's celebrating already. Here comes our next finisher, Caroline Bramwell.'

There they are! Simon and Billy are standing by the side of the finishers' chute, grinning as wildly as I am. Jogging down the chute, I make the most of my moment, high-fiving the boys as I go by. I cross the line! I've made it! I've finished!

As race champion Lucy Gossage hangs the medal around my neck, I am beyond ecstatic. Here I stand as a woman who had been housebound and hospitalised, hugging one of the most amazing female athletes there is after finishing Ironman Staffordshire 70.3. Lucy and

Chrissie Wellington are amazing testimony to dedication to their sport and are the inspiration behind so many people. This moment is surreal.

The first people inside the finishers' chute to congratulate me and give me the biggest hugs are Iron-mums Linda Ogden and Janet Gibson, who have been following my journey for the last 18 months. Brian is next to give me a great big bear hug. He finished not long before me and waited to see me cross the line, whilst Susan had been taken to the medical tent. My ostomy friends and supporters are sitting out in the sunshine too, with all the boys having completed the race as well. What an amazing bunch!

Simon and Billy dash round to the finishers' area for the biggest celebration of all. With their guidance and motivation, I have finished an Ironman race. OK, so they admitted afterwards that they had lied a little about the 50 minutes to cut-off. But, as Simon says, 'It made you run faster.' Thanks guys, you are forgiven! I ring Craig and the kids, who couldn't be here due to having school in the morning, to give them the good news.

Of all the days for me to cross that Ironman finish line, it is ironically Father's Day. I send a special thank-you to my dad, who couldn't be here to watch this.